LIVING
WITH A
SEAL

LIVING WITH A SEAL

31 DAYS TRAINING WITH THE
TOUGHEST MAN ON THE PLANET

JESSE ITZLER

CENTER
STREET

New York Boston Nashville

Center Street
Hachette Book Group
1290 Avenue of the Americas
New York, NY 10104

www.CenterStreet.com

Printed in the United States of America

RRD-C

First edition: November 2015
10 9 8 7 6 5 4 3

Center Street is a division of Hachette Book Group, Inc.
The Center Street name and logo are trademarks of Hachette Book Group, Inc.

The Hachette Speakers Bureau provides a wide range of authors for speaking events. To find out more, go to www.HachetteSpeakersBureau.com or call (866) 376-6591.

The publisher is not responsible for websites (or their content) that are not owned by the publisher.

Library of Congress Cataloging-in-Publication Data has been applied for.

This book is dedicated to my mom and dad, who have been at every game, every event, and every BIG moment in my life. Also, to my wife, who continues to teach me about unwavering support and love. Plus, she has the patience to put up with me.

Disclaimer

The events of this book have been re-created from memory and in some cases have been compressed to convey the substance of what occurred or was said. I tried to keep the time sequence of my experiences in order, but it's possible that events occurred either earlier or later in reality than they do in this story. Although every workout written is true and happened, it's important to note, I'm not recommending you do or try any of the workouts in this book. First off, I don't want anyone to get hurt. Second, who wants to get sued?

Like any activity involving speed, equipment, endurance, and environmental factors, the workouts described in *Living with a SEAL* pose some very serious risks. All readers should take full responsibility for their safety and know their limits. As a trainer, SEAL knew his stuff, and he factored into every single one of his workouts my level of experience, aptitude, training—and how much I could handle.

I kept a detailed diary during my time living with SEAL, which instantly became a blog. It was primarily for friends and family, but as the insanity of my workouts grew, so did my audience. The result is this book.

You will notice in the following pages that the person with whom I trained is referred to only as "SEAL." He asked that I not disclose his name. And he didn't say please.

Contents

Introduction

People ask me why I hired SEAL. One answer is this: When it comes to physical fitness, I tend to be a creature of habit. I guess compared to most people my age, I was in excellent shape and in a great place in my personal life. At the time I was married (still am) to a fantastic woman, and we had our first beautiful eighteen-month-old son (two more since). I began running in 1992, just after I graduated from college. I've missed maybe a handful of days since. I've run eighteen New York City marathons in a row, and it's been the same drill every year. Training schedule—the same. Running route—the same. The store I buy bananas from the day before the race—the same. The Patsy's pizza I order the night before each race—the same.

I like routine.

And routine can be good, especially when it comes to working out. But routine can also be a rut.

Many of us live our lives on autopilot. We do the same thing every day; wake up, go to work, come home, have dinner. Repeat. I found myself drifting in that direction. It was as if my cruise control settings had been set and I wasn't improving. I wanted to get off it; I wanted to shake things up in a big way. My Central Park West life and SEAL's nomadic take-no-prisoners life merging (or I should say, colliding) for a period of time was what I needed. It was unexpected, it was unique. It was insane (okay, I admit it), but research shows that stepping out of our routine in life is great for the body and spirit...the brain too. Mix it up! Do the outrageous; think out of the box. Life is short, why not? As SEAL says, "This ain't a dress rehearsal, bitch."

While this is a story about our month together, it's just as much a story about two people that had to step outside of their comfort zones. SEAL and me. He was as uncomfortable with doormen, chefs, and drivers as I was with sleeping in a chair and intentionally waking up in the middle of the night to run in the worst possible conditions. His no rhyme or reason approach to our workout schedule actually brought a lot of clarity into my life.

SEAL had something I wanted, but I just wasn't sure what it was. And I wanted to find out. Do you remember Mr. Miyagi from *The Karate Kid*? He had a very unorthodox approach to training. Daniel LaRusso, played by Ralph Macchio, wants to learn martial arts, but Mr. Miyagi starts him off with menial chores to help him. And Daniel unknowingly develops the defensive blocks through muscle memory, but what he eventually learns is a lot more than martial arts. That's kind of what I was looking for when I asked SEAL to move in and train me. I wanted to train my body, but also my mind and spirit. The difference was I wasn't training for protection or a trophy. And I had already gotten the girl. I just wanted to get better.

I've also always had an unorthodox approach to business and life in general. It's served me well. I don't believe in résumés in the traditional sense, I believe in life résumés. Do more. Create memories. Only when looking back on my successes and failures am I able to connect the dots. I could have never predicted or planned to go from being a rapper on MTV in the 1990s to eventually owning and operating my own private jet company. My normal has always been abnormal.

I don't know if I was thinking about my mortality, or fretting over how many more peak years I had left, or anything like that. I just felt that now was as good a time as any to shake things up. You know, to break up that *same* routine.

I believe the best ideas are the ones you don't spend too much time thinking through. My time with SEAL was no different and I got a lot more than I bargained for. Most of my successes in life have come from learning how to be comfortable with being uncomfortable. Like I said, I just want to get better.

Every day do something that makes you uncomfortable.

—SEAL

PROLOGUE

SEAL moved into my home to train me in December 2010. That winter went on to be one of the snowiest on record. Airports closed. Trains were delayed. A nor'easter dropped more than twenty inches of snow on New York City in one day. The winds were so strong they pushed the falling snow into drifts that measured up to four feet. City bus drivers abandoned their vehicles in the middle of the streets. So did regular drivers. Plows couldn't remove the snow for days. I was sure my mission with SEAL would be compromised. But that was before I knew him.

DAY 1

The Arrival

I'm trained to disappear.
—SEAL

New York City
14°
0638

I pour oatmeal into a bowl, fill the pot with water, light the stove, and set the timer. I click play on the remote and position Lazer, my eighteen-month-old son, so he can see his *Baby Einstein* video. I peek into the guest room to make sure the bed is made. My son is giggling, which comforts me. I check on my wife, Sara, who's still sleeping, and then recheck the guest room to make sure it's shipshape, or whatever the heck they say in the Navy. I hear the timer go off. I cut up some bananas and pour honey on them. I look at the clock on the microwave: 6:38 a.m.

ETA: twenty-two minutes.

I'm filled with nervous energy.

I sit with my son, feed him breakfast, and watch the rest of *Baby Einstein*. The bananas are still in my bowl. I'm not hungry. I go into the bathroom and look at myself in the mirror. I push my hair back with my hands. I grin at my reflection to check my teeth. They're clean.

I go back to the living room.

I do as many push-ups as I can: twenty-two.

I look at the clock: 6:44 a.m.

What if he has trouble getting a cab? Does a guy like him even take a cab? Maybe he's going to run to my house. The plane might be delayed? He could've changed his mind? Maybe I should call. What am I talking about? The guy's probably parachuted into foreign countries; he has to know how to get to my house on time. Right?

But he *NEVER* asked for my address, *NEVER* inquired what to bring. He *wouldn't* give me his flight information and *didn't* request a car service. *NOTHING*. In fact, the only thing the man said was:

"I arrive at oh seven hundred." That's military time for 7:00 a.m.

❖ ❖ ❖

I first saw "SEAL" at a twenty-four-hour relay race in San Diego. After several marathons, this was my first "ultra." I was on a team of six ultra-marathoners who would each take turns running twenty-minute legs. The objective: Run more miles than every other team in twenty-four hours.

There were teams registered from all over the country.

You know, friends coming together to test themselves physically and mentally. SEAL, however, didn't have a team. He didn't have friends. He was running the entire race... himself.

The event was low budget, really low budget. The entire course was set around a one-mile loop in an unlit parking lot near the San Diego Zoo. It was unsupported, meaning you bring your own supplies. Whatever you needed, you were responsible for.

My team and I flew in the night before to get ready. When we got there we walked the course and mapped out our strategy. Before we went to sleep, we laid out our race gear and supplies so we were ready to go when we woke up. Water. Gatorade. Bananas. PowerBars. Band-Aids. We were ready.

Before the race, we stretched in a small circle on the grass. I was nervous and excited, but I couldn't help notice the guy ten feet away. To say he stood out would be an understatement. For starters, he was the only African-American in the race. Secondly, he weighed over 260 pounds whereas most of the other runners weighed between 140 and 165 pounds. Third, whereas everyone else was talkative and friendly, this guy seemed pissed. I mean he looked very angry.

He just sat there all by himself in a folding chair with his arms crossed waiting for the race to start. No stretching, no prep, no fancy shoes, and no teammates. No smiling. He just sat quietly with a don't-fuck-with-me expression on his face. His supplies for twenty-four hours: one box of crackers and water. That's it. He laid them out next to his chair.

The guy was a cross between a gladiator and the G.I. Joe action hero my son has, but life size. He looked indestructible. Battle tested. Dangerous. Alone. Determined.

Even the way he spit was scary. If he hit you with it, it likely would leave a scar. He was intimidating. Physically, the man looked like someone sprayed muscle paint all over his body. Ripped. Flawless.

Once the race started, in between our individual legs of running, we stretched and stayed hydrated to avoid injury, and applied plenty of Vaseline. As a friend of mine likes to say: "Brother, ultras are chafey." But as the race continued and I cheered on my teammates, I couldn't help but keep tabs on the guy who was running alone. Who *was* this guy?

There was magnetism to his fury. Underneath his scowl I sensed something I couldn't quite put my finger on. Maybe it was a sense of honor or integrity. Or purpose. Yeah, that's it. He ran with a sense of purpose that I couldn't quite comprehend. He ran as though lives depended on it, like he was running into a burning house to save someone, a kitten or an old woman. With each stride he took it seemed like he was creating mini-earthquakes beneath his feet, but at all times his form was perfect, his eyes locked in a stare, a focus that was diamond-tip PRECISE. He just ran…checked his splits on his watch…and ran for a hundred miles straight.

When the twenty-four-hour race was over, I was cooked. My thighs were so tight I could barely walk a yard. As my teammates and I slowly gathered our extra sneakers, lawn chairs, and personal belongings, I noticed him again, this massive, two-hundred-plus-pound block of carbon steel, being helped to the parking lot by a woman (whom I would later find out was his wife), looking like he just survived a plane crash.

I concluded two things:

1. I had never seen anyone like this.
2. I had to meet him.

Back home, after some investigating and some Googling, I was able to ascertain a few pertinent things about him, including the fact that he was a Navy SEAL, a highly decorated Navy SEAL at that. Then I tracked down a contact number and called him cold. He was on the West Coast.

This is a habit I have. When I see or read about someone interesting, I call them up and basically ask them to be my friend. My wife says it reminds her of middle school when you hand someone a note and ask, "Do you want to be my friend? Check yes or no." Well, I guess I never outgrew that phase.

"Yeah?" he answered.

"Is this SEAL?"

"That depends on who's asking," he said.

I hadn't experienced these kind of nerves since I called Sue my senior year in high school to ask her to the prom. I started talking about the race and babbling on, until halfway through my rap I realized that I sounded like someone I would've hung up on. In fact, I wasn't completely sure he hadn't hung up—there was dead silence coming from his end of the phone.

This was way worse than the call to Sue.

"Hello?" I asked.

"Yeah."

"Just give me fifteen minutes to propose something to you in person," I said finally. "I'm in New York City but can fly out tomorrow."

Silence.

"Hello?"

Silence.

"SEAL?"

Silence.

Finally: "You wanna come out…it's on you," he said.

Twenty-four hours later I was in California.

We met in a local restaurant in San Diego. After some small talk, which consisted of me talking and him saying nothing in response, I asked him to move into my house to train me.

He stared at me with cold, flat eyes. I couldn't tell if he thought I was nuts or if he was figuring out if I was worth his time. He was sizing me up.

One minute passed. Then another.

"Okay, I'll do it with one condition," he said in a tone that was slightly motivational in a psychopathic drill sergeant way. "You do everything I say."

"Yes."

"And that means EVERYTHING."

"Okay."

"I can wake you at any time; I can push you to any extreme."

"Ummm."

"NOTHING is off limits. NOTHING."

"Well..."

"By the time we're done you'll be able to do a thousand push-ups in a day."

"A thousand?"

This wasn't going to be anything like the prom, I thought.

* * *

At exactly 7:00 a.m. there's a knock on my door.

He has *NO luggage. NO suitcases. NO expression.* In spite of the fact that it's December and it's *freezing* out, he's wearing *NO coat. NO hat. NO gloves.* And there's NO greeting.

He simply says, "You ready?"

That's it? No warm-up pitch? No "nice to see you again"? No "it's cold out, huh?" Maybe something nice and easy, right down the middle? Instead, I get a Mariano Rivera cut fastball.

"I'm so glad you're here," I say. "Anything you need, please feel free to help yourself. Make yourself at home. Our home is your home."

"Nah, bro! Not at all, this is *your* home. I don't have a home."

I laugh.

SEAL doesn't laugh.

"It was only an expression," I answer. "Make yourself at home, that's an expression."

"I don't operate in expressions, dude. I operate in actions. That needs to be clear immediately," he says. "Understand?"

"Okay."

"Huh?"

"Yes . . . sir?"

"I'm trained to disappear. You won't EVER even know when I'm here."

"Okay."

"Ah'ite. Let's get into this shit. Meet me here in nine minutes. And don't bring your cowfuck expressions."

Cowfuck?

I change into my standard cold-weather workout gear, which consists of two sweatshirts, two hats, and gloves. I walk back out to the front door, where SEAL is already standing, looking at his watch. It's fourteen degrees out and nippy. He's wearing shorts, a T-shirt, and a knit hat. Nothing else.

"Man, I may need to borrow some gloves," says SEAL.

"You *may* need gloves?"

"Yeah, or some kinda mittens or some shit like that."

"That's it. Only gloves?"

"That's it."

"It's fourteen degrees outside," I say.

"To you it's fourteen degrees 'cause you're telling yourself it's fourteen degrees!"

"No. It really is. It's fourteen degrees. Like that's the real actual temperature outside. It says so on my computer."

SEAL pauses for a moment like I may have disappointed him. "On your computer, huh?"

He begins to laugh, but it's a haunting laugh, like the Count on *Sesame Street*.

"The temperature is what you think it is, bro, not what your computer thinks it is. If you think it's fourteen degrees, then it's fourteen degrees. Personally, I'm looking at it like it's in the mid-fifties."

Rather than argue—after all, we're still just getting to know each other—I just say: "Got it."

"You ever spent any time in freezing water, Jesse?" SEAL asks.

I'm thinking to myself, Like on purpose? But I respond with a "no."

"Well, is it freezing? OR is your *mind* just saying it's freezing? Which is it?" He laughs again. "Control your *mind*, Jesse."

"Got it." (I'm going to have to put that on the to-do list: *Control mind.*)

"Exactly. Enjoy this shit. If you want it to be seventy and sunny...it's seventy and sunny. Just run. The elements are in your mind. I don't ever check the temperature when I run. Who gives a fuck what the temperature on the computer says? The computer isn't out there running, is it?"

He's got me there, but instead of saying "got it" again, I try to keep the banter going.

"Does that work the same way in heat? I mean, if it's ninety-five degrees outside, can you make it snow in your mind?"

"Nah, man, it's a one-way system, bro. Cold to hot only. When it's hot outside...it's just fucking hot!"

If one of my friends tried to give me the same logic, I'd laugh, but coming from SEAL's mouth, I almost believe him.

However, I can feel the draft coming from our windows and I don't care what SEAL says—it really is fourteen degrees outside.

"Well, then, what's the strategy in the heat?"

"In extreme heat, it's a totally different mind-set, bro. You have to get medieval. Embrace it! Grind it out. Think about how others are suffering. Enjoy the pain."

"Yours or theirs?" I ask.

SEAL levels me with his stare.

"Both," he says. Then SEAL nods at me, the signal that it's "go" time.

We head to Central Park and run six miles at a 9:20-mile pace. I think SEAL wants to feel me out. Although I am an experienced marathoner, I was never a fast runner. I can run at a seven-minute pace, but I prefer not to. I like to take my time running; my pace is more the you-should-be-able-to-talk-to-a-friend-while-running pace. It's more enjoyable. I'm way more of an endurance guy than a sprint guy. I find that endurance running is more of a mental challenge than a physical challenge, and I'm pretty good at blocking out the pain and boredom of long runs.

This pace suits me well. I think to myself, I can do this.

An hour later...

After a warm shower and quickly returning some work emails, I give SEAL a quick tour of our apartment. We live at 15 Central Park West on the Upper West Side of Manhattan.

The building has been written and blogged about as a famous New York City building and also been featured for its amazing views, architecture, and residents. Many of the world's top CEOs, athletes, and entertainers live in the building.

I convinced Sara two years ago we should move in because the building had a pool. "We can swim every day, honey." Well, here we are two years later. We bought the apartment but we have not been in the pool once.

Although my wife and I don't consider ourselves to be "fancy," the building sure is. In fact, when we first moved in, the elevator concierge (not the elevator operator; the elevator *concierge*) told me to get off of the elevator because the elevators are "only for residents." I guess I didn't look the part of resident in my ski hat and shorts.

I start the tour by showing SEAL how to use the remotes for the television. I figure that is something a guest who is staying with us for over a month will want to know, right?

"This is how you turn it on," I say, pointing to the power button.

"We won't be watching much TV," he says, interrupting me.

"Okay then…Moving on," I say.

I set the remote down and then lead him over to the kitchen. If we aren't going to be watching television, then we certainly will be eating, I assume. I pull out the first drawer.

"So this is where all the forks, spoons, and knives are," I say.

"I won't be using your utensils," he says.

Huh? I close the drawer.

Maybe I'll have more luck in the laundry room.

As I am about to show him how to use the washer and dryer, he interrupts me again and says, "Yo, man, you can skip all this tour shit. Just tell me how to get to the gym."

Okay. The tour is officially over and we head to the gym.

For the first time I can see SEAL's front teeth as a smile starts to form. He is ecstatic; I can see the change in his expression just from walking inside of the gym. It's almost like watching *The Wizard of Oz* for the first time when you see the screen go from black and white to color. It's a whole new world. He walks over to the pull-up bar, jumps up, grabs the bar, and hangs. He starts to swing and swing some more and swing until he finally jumps off. I guess he approves because his smile has grown.

"This is perfect. You ready?" he asks.

"For what?"

"Your pulls."

"You mean like right now?"

"Give me ten. All the way down and all the way up. Let's see where your pull-up game is at."

I jump up and grab the bar and pull my two hundred pounds of body weight up until my chin is over the bar. "One."

I go down. When I get to number eight, I start kicking my legs around frantically to try to get some momentum. I need to get my chin over this damn bar, but I can't. I drop to the floor. SEAL tells me to take a forty-five-second break and do it again.

Forty-five seconds later I jump back up and grab the bar. I've never been good at doing pull-ups. In fact, I hate doing them. Somehow I manage to squeak out six more before I drop back to the ground. This time I think for good. SEAL tells me to take another forty-five seconds and then do it again.

Another forty-five seconds go by and this time I'm able to get three solid pull-ups in before I drop to the ground. Each time I'm dropping, my legs give out a little more. That's seventeen pull-ups. I'm *done*. I'm literally maxed out. I don't think I have ever done seventeen pull-ups so fast, or *ever*, for that matter. I grab my left bicep with my right hand and my right bicep with my left hand and squeeze. It feels like there are nails in my biceps.

"Seventeen! Cool, that's my max number. I didn't think I could even do that. Amazing! Let's head back upstairs."

As I start to look up, SEAL is staring at me with a blank expression...deadpan. "We're going to stay here until you do a hundred."

WHAT?

"I can't do a hundred. That's impossible," I say.

"You better find a way," he says to me like a father might tell his son to clean his bedroom. "You got a shitty-ass attitude."

I do one and drop to the floor.

I walk around the gym trying to delay the inevitable. My arms sag at my sides and SEAL watches me. I can't procrastinate any longer. I return to the pull-up bar. I do another one and drop to the ground. I take another lap around the gym

and I'm back to the pull-up bar. I drop. Lap...Pull-up...
Drop...Lap...Pull-up...Drop...

Ninety minutes later I'm on ninety-seven.

Training is definitely under way.

Workout totals: 6 miles and 100 pull-ups

No Novocain

I like to sit back and enjoy the pain. I earned it.
—SEAL

I grew up on Long Island in Roslyn, New York, with two older sisters and a brother. I was the youngest by five years. As suburban as you can get, Roslyn has developments of houses that all are pretty much the same with connected backyards that were patrolled by an army of kids my age. My mom owned a cowbell. I could be six or seven houses away and I'd hear my mom's bell calling me home. I was trained like a cow; it was slightly embarrassing. The rule was: Do your homework and you can go outside, but when you hear the bell, you'd better come home and you'd better be home in five minutes. My mom was the most unconditionally loving mom, but my mom was a hard-ass. Nobody messed with her. I've never heard her curse, but she has this look that she'd give you: her go-to move. Silence. It got me every time.

My mom was also something of a dichotomy when it came to traditional child healthcare. On one hand, she'd let me eat cheeseburgers, bacon, ice cream, and Oreo cookies, whatever I wanted, and all at once; but she was freaked out by X-ray machines, fluoride, and Novocain. She didn't think there had been enough research and testing done on certain things in the 1970s, and she didn't want me to be the lab rat. I got my first X-ray only after they invented that big lead vest they put on you, and she thought fluoride was just the most toxic thing. Not having X-rays and fluoride in my life was easy to take. What was hard was no Novocain.

My dentist's name was Henry Schmitzer, and his office was about a forty-five-minute drive from our house. I guess he was the only dentist my mom could find who would drill a kid's mouth without an anesthetic. Henry might have been Laurence Olivier's inspiration for the character he played in *Marathon Man*.

So while all of my friends were getting gassed-up, pain-free, and lollipoped visits to their dentists around the corner, I'd be sitting in the back of the car for forty-five minutes, staring out the window, sweating, thinking…we are actually driving out of our way for this shit. That sound, and smell, like burning bone, of the drill. The anticipation was grueling, to say the least. It was a full-on event for me. The walk from the parking lot to the office always sparked thoughts and temptations to just run away as fast as I could. But my mother would give me a sympathetic smile as she held the door for me to go inside—she really believed she was doing the best for me. .

Inside, Schmitzer the motherfucker, would start drilling my mouth. (I'm literally holding my mouth as I'm writing this.) The taste of that fire, the sound, the excruciating pain, and my mouth would be sore forever. It was crazy. You'd think that would have been motivation to brush better, but it always seemed like I had at least one cavity every checkup.

My dad was basically the complete opposite from Mom, in a go-with-the-flow type of way. He owned a plumbing supply store in Mineola and worked six days a week (a half day on Saturday). Even with all the time he invested at work, he was a hands-on dad. He showed up for every game, every event, and made it a point to be home for family dinner every night.

At home he was like a mad scientist—he had a workshop in his basement, and that was his spot. He wasn't into watching sports or hanging out with friends, he liked to invent. When the movie *Back to the Future* came out and "Doc" created the Flux Capacitor...I was like, *"That's my dad!!"*

I remember one time in elementary school when I had to make a diorama. The assignment was simple: Take a shoebox and create a replica of your own house. Well, by the time my dad "helped out," my diorama had running water and electricity. I kid you not. You could also push a button and the little garage door on the diorama would open.

I definitely think I got my creativity from my dad. And as far as I know he's pro-Novocain, but unfortunately he wasn't the one driving me to the dentist.

The part of me that would grow up to hire a Navy SEAL, that came from Mom.

DAY 2

Nature's Gatorade

I'm the surprise-or. Not the surprise-ee.
—SEAL

New York City to Boston
20° to 16°
0700

I had a hard time sleeping last night. It's a combination of nerves and excitement mixed in with the fact that my biceps are jacked up from the pull-ups. They are sore to the touch. I don't think they moved once from the ninety-degree flexed position they were stuck in all night.

As far as nerves go, I am unusually nervous right now. It's not the typical type of nerves someone might get from having to go on a job interview or something like that, but it's nervousness in the sense that I don't want to disappoint SEAL by not being able to do the workouts. This anxiety started to build before he ever arrived. And the thought of not wanting to get hurt is playing like background music in my head. It's a little like the nerves I feel before a marathon. There's a level of uncertainty of what will and might happen. Plus, the way SEAL expected me to do a hundred pull-ups yesterday was borderline certifiable. And he refused to leave the gym until they were all done.

It freaked me out.

Anyway, before we went to bed last night, SEAL told me to set my alarm clock for 0630 (6:30 a.m.) in preparation for a run at 0700 (7:00 a.m.)...SHARP.

Well, there was no alarm clock needed because at 6:00 a.m. I hear someone walking around the foyer of the apartment. Not tiptoeing, but making what feels like intentional noise to wake me up. I hear an excessive loud fake coughing...the slamming of the front door...and music being turned up extra loud.

What an asshole.

I grab two sweatshirts, two hats, and gloves. SEAL is in the same summer attire as yesterday with the addition of some old gloves I lent him. We head out.

As we walk by the front desk, I can tell the doormen are curious as to who SEAL is. I thought I overheard one of them asking the other if he was Jerry Rice, the football great.

"Nah, this guy is way bigger than Jerry Rice," the other said.

We run the same loop of Central Park as we did yesterday at the same nine-minute-mile pace. There is *no* talking. There is *no* joking. There is *no* communication. I'm not so sure this guy wants to be my friend...and I'm not so sure I now want to be his.

My arms hurt like hell from the pull-ups, but I don't say anything. I just keep stride. I have run long distances in my life, but when I'm not training on a daily basis, a six-mile run is a pain in the ass. It's *long* and definitely can be boring. No matter how you slice it, six miles is going to take me fifty to sixty minutes. That's a long time to be running.

Any runner will tell you that some days a run can fly by and be enjoyable. And sometimes that same exact run on the same exact path feels like torture and is excruciatingly slow. Today the clock seems to be ticking particularly slowly. Maybe it's the awkwardness of running with a stranger. It's very odd running with someone you don't know and who doesn't speak. The silence is very uncomfortable. It's like running with someone who speaks a language you don't understand...except this someone is very intimidating and will be living with you for another thirty days. Whatever it is, this run feels twice as long as it did the last time I ran it.

When we get home I make a quick shake, shower, and head to work.

Three hours later...

I haven't told SEAL that today I have to fly to Boston for a business meeting around noon. But I have good reason for the trip. I recently started a company called the 100 Mile Group. I'm fairly good at identifying trends and predicting the next big thing. The 100 Mile Group is set up to take advantage of that. If I find a product or service that I know customers will want and I have authentic passion for it, then our company will invest, market, or launch it.

Our first product is a new brand called Zico Coconut Water. As a runner I am well aware of the amazing hydrating qualities of coconut water and am convinced the category is going to take off. I had also noticed that every four years or so, a new, natural health drink would hit the market and explode off the shelves. Pomegranate juice had just stormed the castle—everywhere you looked there was an ad for the stuff. I believed coconut water was next.

Initially I looked into importing coconut water from overseas and having a go at it myself. After trips to Jamaica and Brazil, I quickly realized I would be much better off partnering with an existing brand and helping them grow their business.

I was introduced to Mark Rampolla, the founder of Zico Coconut Water, that summer. Zico was a small company at the time with about $5 million in sales, but my Spidey senses told me they were onto something, plus I really liked Mark. I ended up partnering with the company and simultaneously brokered a deal with Coca-Cola where they came in as a minority partner.

Coca-Cola had recently established a division called VEB, Venturing & Emerging Brands. This is the branch of Coke that looks for the next billion-dollar brand and partners with them during their early growth period. They were responsible for acquiring Honest Tea, Illy Coffee, and other hot brands. My friend Lance Collins had founded Fuze and just sold it to Coke. He introduced me to the president of the division, and after several trips to Atlanta we formed a three-way partnership: Zico, the 100 Mile Group, and Coca-Cola. Coke retained an option to acquire the whole company based on certain sales triggers. Zico is starting to take off, so this is a big meeting for me.

I eventually tell SEAL we have to go to Boston for the

meeting. I totally forgot to give him the heads-up, but I'm sure he'll understand—it's business.

"This is some bullshit, Jesse. I'm gonna do it, but this is some pure cow BULLSHIT. No more motherfuckin' surprises, Jesse. I'm the surprise-or, not the surprise-ee. I'm not playin'. NO MORE FUCKING SURPRISES. We can't deviate." He is livid.

"I promise we'll be back by seven p.m. tonight to train," I say, hoping to smooth over his disappointment. He agrees, but in my mind I'm thinking, What real choice does he have? I have to work, right?

It's noon. We go straight to the airport from my office. There's no need to stop by my apartment and pack because I'm positive we'll be back in time for our evening workout. I have an extra pair of shorts and a T-shirt under my desk at work so I grab them...just in case.

The fact that I'm going to be meeting with Boston Celtic and basketball legend Kevin Garnett does very little to impress SEAL. This is my first time meeting Garnett and I'm looking forward to it. I've been good friends with his sports agent for a while, and I'd heard Garnett was a fan of Zico, even though he's officially an endorser of Gatorade. And Garnett is a fitness freak.

In the off season Garnett lives in Malibu. But Garnett does not technically have an off season because as soon as the season ends, he gets right to training. He prides himself on working out early and often. "I like my feet to be the first footprints in the sand," he's said many times. I love the guy's intensity and focus on wellness. I think he'll be a perfect fit as an investor and endorser for Zico. Plus, it would be huge for us to lure him away from Gatorade, and I believe his contract with them is coming up for renewal. Needless to say, I'm excited for this meeting.

On the jet, I buckle my seat belt as tight as I can and point the air valve directly at me. Then I pull the shade down over the window. I've never been the greatest flyer (which is ironic because I started a private jet company). As part of my superstition, I go through a kind of preflight checklist every time I get on a plane. I say a prayer, put on Carole King, and click my heels three times. And this time I'm glad I do. To say the takeoff is bumpy doesn't capture the experience. It's a nauseating roller coaster. The plane is being tossed around like a pinball from side to side.

In between the free falls, I glance over at SEAL. He's still in the same running shorts and T-shirt he ran in this a.m., and he's reading *Sports Illustrated*. I'm not sure SEAL realizes we even took off yet as he casually flips the pages of his magazine. He's unfazed.

Twenty minutes into the flight a beeping noise chimes indicating a warning and the buckle-your-seat-belt sign illuminates. The pilot instructs the flight attendants to "return to their seats and stop service" as the turbulence is so severe. I'm flipped out and have convinced myself we are going down. Beads of sweat are pouring down my forehead and my palms are drenched. But SEAL, he doesn't so much as flinch. He's just reading. Casually flipping the pages and yawning.

Finally we are wheels down in Boston. I'm ecstatic that we are on the ground in one piece.

SEAL couldn't give two shits. He turns to me and says, "Great flight."

1600

We walk into the conference room of the Boston Celtics' practice facility and there's Kevin Garnett, his agent, and one of his financial guys. Kevin is much taller than I anticipated, and he is super ripped. The guy looks way more muscular and intimidating in person. He had just finished a three-hour practice and was showered up and ready to discuss business.

We're led to a large room that overlooks the court where the team's executives sit when they watch practice. I'm feeling pretty good. I enjoy putting people and products that I believe in together and am quite at ease in this kind of meeting, so going in my confidence level is on high.

"Hey, Kevin, man, Jesse Itzler…" I go to shake Garnett's hand, which is the size of a Hamburger Helper hand, but I realize he's not looking at me. He's looking at SEAL.

"And this is SEAL," I say.

SEAL nods, then Garnett does. It's like a silent standoff— two gunslingers in the Wild West evaluating each other.

"I hired a Navy SEAL to live with me for a month or so," I say to explain. "You know, to train me. To shake some shit up in my life."

Garnett's eyebrows arch as if I'm the first person to bring a Navy SEAL to a business meeting with him.

"Is it okay if he joins us for the meeting?"

I hand Garnett a Zico Coconut Water, smile, and jump right into my pitch: "If Mother Nature went into the sports drink business, Zico would be her Gatorade…"

"How many miles you run a day?" Garnett asks SEAL, finally breaking the silence that has been building between them.

"Depends," SEAL says with a shrug.

"Do weights or resistance training?"

"Yes and no," SEAL says.

"Anaerobic threshold?"

"Body composition?"

"Maximum heart rate?"

"Your VO2?"

Garnett fires the questions and SEAL parries them back. It's not a gunfight, it's more like Garnett is in the quarter-finals at the U.S. Open in Flushing, Queens, and SEAL is playing badminton at a cookout.

Hours pass. Not once do we talk about Zico. I'm just sitting there. We talk about workouts. Or rather *they* talk about workouts. I can tell that SEAL is digging Garnett. There is some kind of mutual warrior vibe going on that they are connecting with. I'm picking it up too, but I'm not on the same warrior vibe radio station as them.

Weather starts to roll in. The meeting goes on, and on, *and on*!

"Ah'ite," Garnett finally says, signaling the meeting's over.

What about Zico? I'm wondering.

Garnett and SEAL turn and look at me like I've just magically reappeared. They give each other a bear hug and we say our good-byes.

Finally Garnett turns to me. "It's as simple as this, yo. Whatever you motherfuckers do," Garnett says, "I want in."

2000

I give SEAL a high fist bump as we walk out of the building. The euphoria quickly turns into fear as we walk out into a full-fledged snow squall. This isn't good, I think to myself. This is what SEAL might refer to as a surprise, but this one's on Mother Nature—not me. We don't even attempt to go to the airport, and I find us a hotel near the Boston Garden. It's getting late as we check into our rooms. I'm tired and need to rest. Maybe I'll rent a movie and order room service. Just as I lie down on the bed I hear a knock.

"Let's go," the voice says through the door. "Meet in the lobby in ten minutes."

"But it's freezing and snowing."

"Ten minutes."

"But we ran already this morning."

"Ten minutes."

"But I don't have anything warm?"

Eight minutes later I get off the elevator in the lobby. SEAL is ready. He's waiting at the front desk. He looks at me like I'm late when in actuality I'm two minutes early. It's our second run of the day, and the temperature keeps dropping. I'm in shorts, a T-shirt, a hat, and the sweatshirt I wore to the meeting. That's it. It's eighteen degrees outside and we run along the Boston waterfront. It's bitter cold, windy with a misty snow. I really *don't* want to be out here, but I have no choice. I'm freezing my ass off. I want to be in my hotel room ordering room service and watching the snow from behind

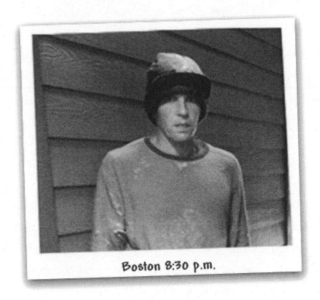

Boston 8:30 p.m.

my window. Plus, all I really want to do is think about the next steps with Zico and Garnett while it's fresh on my mind.

I try to break down the Garnett meeting with SEAL and discuss the win.

"That meeting was awesome," I say.

No response.

"You think his financial guy dug it?"

No response.

"What did you think of his financial guy anyway?"

No response. About one minute later SEAL finally says, "Motherfucker, it's KG's show." I'll leave it at that.

I'm not sure exactly what body of water we are running next to this evening, but I assume it's the Charles River. I have *nothing* to base that off of other than the fact that it's the only river I know of in Boston. Whether I'm right or wrong, I visualize the river filled with college kids rowing on a hot day. I'm not sure SEAL is visualizing anything. He is just staring straight ahead as if he is anticipating an ambush. But no enemies appear.

When we get back to the hotel, my fingertips are frozen. I go to Google "frostbite" on my laptop, but I can't work the keypad. We just logged six more miles. That's twelve for the day and eighteen so far.

I throw my wet clothes in the bathtub, lay my sweatshirt out on the heater in the room to dry, and call Sara to check in. Whenever I'm on the road, it's tough being away from my wife and son (but a call always warms me up). It's 9:30 p.m. real time and she's not picking up. It just keeps ringing.

Sara likes to go to bed early. It's been like that since the day I met her in 2006 at a poker tournament in Las Vegas.

Sara was a customer of mine at Marquis Jet, the private jet company I co-founded in 2001. Our partner, NetJets, was hosting a poker tournament, and we were allocated only forty seats at the tables. We had three thousand–plus customers at that point, and picking forty was hard to do. Every sales rep got to submit a list of four or five clients they thought were worthy of being invited, and then my partner Kenny and I would choose one person from each region to invite.

My Georgia sales rep called me and said she had a young businesswoman who she thought should get a ticket. The rep then emailed me a photo of her. The picture was a headshot of a pretty blonde with an apple on her head. *What?* I was intrigued. She was a cutie! So I told the rep not to send any other applications my way and to go ahead and invite her, the girl with the apple on her head.

The night of the tournament, about fifteen of us went out to dinner, and the woman with the apple on her head was in the group. Then, thirty minutes into the dinner, she said it was past her bedtime and was going back to her room. I looked at my phone. It was 9:30 p.m. Who goes to bed at 9:30 at night in Vegas? What an odd bird, I thought. Two years later I was married to that odd bird.

My call goes into voicemail and I leave a message. Since it's past 9:00 p.m., Sara must be sound asleep, and it's time for me to call it a night. With all of the weather delays, I assume the airport will be backed up and I want to get there early in the morning.

Workout totals: 12 miles in freezing rain

DAY 3

My Nuts

You need to feel the pace.
—SEAL

Boston
28°
0500

The hotel phone is ringing. What time is it? I didn't request a wake-up call. Obviously it's SEAL, so I roll over in bed and pick it up.

"It's go time" is the first thing I hear.

Yesterday, SEAL told me he wanted me to run six miles in the morning and three miles at night for the first three days he's here to build my "base."

Three days to build a base? That sounds ridiculous. Doesn't it take months to build a base?

Anyway, I wasn't expecting to be in Boston overnight, so I have no extra clothes to change into, plus my clothing from last night is still soaking wet and cold from the snow and sweat. Before we head down I meet SEAL in the hallway between our rooms to discuss a little issue I have.

"SEAL, I have a problem," I say to him. "I didn't bring any extra underwear."

"So what?"

"I can't run without underwear."

"Nah, bro, you can't run without legs. It's on."

So I throw on my freezing wet clothes from last night. I'm cold and miserable before I even head out. My underwear is so wet that I can't put it on, so I go "commando" style.

We meet in the lobby.

Today's pace is faster than last night's, like a minute per mile faster. And somebody forgot to give the sun a wake-up call because it's still pitch black out. We dart in and out of the headlights of incoming traffic like inmates fleeing the yard in a prison break. We zig, horns beep, and we zag, horns blast. I'm just trying to keep pace.

Apparently SEAL prefers to run on the street facing traffic and as close to the moving cars as possible. Like why not run on the sidewalk? Why are we on the street? The answer is I'm not really sure why. Maybe he likes the adrenaline rush. I don't. I prefer to run on a quiet street where there's no exhaust and cars aren't coming within an inch of killing me! Whatever the reason, he insists on running that way.

There's a sidewalk two feet from us that we can easily jump on. It may even be *for* runners. It's clean, empty, safe, and appealing. SEAL ignores it. We stay on the street narrowly avoiding cars and jumping over potholes. It's driving me crazy. WHY CAN'T HE GO ON THE SIDEWALK?

After twenty minutes or so, SEAL has only said two words to me.

"Stay close."

At about three miles into our six-mile run, it's time to turn around to run back to the hotel, so we do. The sun begins to peek through. It's 5:30 a.m. I'm getting better at dodging traffic, but I still don't like it.

It's on the route home when I begin to realize something isn't quite right. It's my nuts. They're starting to rub against the fabric of my shorts because I'm running without under-wear. It's not a pleasurable feeling.

Without breaking stride I put my right hand on my balls, pull my fingers out of my shorts, and look...Blood! Con-firmed. It's my nuts. My balls are bleeding from the friction. Jesus!

"SEAL, my nuts are bleeding."

"Who gives a fuck about your tiny nuts?" he says.

We keep pace.

About a mile later I realize I don't recognize anything. The buildings...the trees...nothing on the way back to the hotel looks familiar. This is not the way we came.

"Sorry, man, but nothing looks familiar. I assume it's impossible that you could get lost?" I manage to ask in between gasps. "Not with your training?"

He glares at me. "Ranger school, bro...No chance."

After forty-eight minutes of running, his watch beeps for the sixth time indicating we've hit the six-mile mark, but no hotel in sight. I'm thinking three miles out, three miles back...Run should be over, right? Come on, man. My nuts are fucking bloody.

At 8.3 miles, we finally find the hotel.

I'm pissed off about the extra mileage. SEAL is satisfied. It's like he thinks he got extra credit or something. The second we get inside, SEAL pulls out his training log and jots down a recap of the workout. Date. Time. Pace. Mileage, etc. He writes so small he has the details of his whole year of workouts on two pages. I walk bow-legged across the lobby. It hurts. I wonder if the concierge can help with bleeding nuts.

"Ranger school, bro."

Three hours later...

I call SEAL's room and tell him we'd better get to the airport.

"Roger that," he says.

It's 9:00 a.m. We're stuck for hours at Logan. Nothing's flying. I make some calls. I'm happy thinking over the way the Garnett meeting went down. I read some magazines. I walk around. I make some more calls. SEAL just sits there, staring straight ahead. He doesn't move off the chair. He doesn't go to the bathroom. I'm not even sure he blinks. He's just staring.

I look over in the direction of what he's staring at to identify it. I follow his eyes to a blank brick wall. There is nothing there. I look back at him to double check I'm lining up his sight line correctly. And again, it takes me to the brick wall. He is just staring. Like the stone lion in front of the New York Public Library.

SEAL has two gears: idle and full out. But his idle isn't like normal idle at all; it's more like the moment between ignition and blastoff. I get the feeling around him that things could get hairy quickly. And yet I also have a feeling of absolute safety around him. I don't mean my own personal safety, though there's that too. I mean like national defense safety.

For three more hours I pace, eat, shop, and read. SEAL just stares. We finally board our flight.

Still Day 3. That night.

Thankfully, the flight is much smoother than the ride to Boston. I am able to close my eyes for the fifty minutes to New York, and it feels like I am in a full REM cycle. I'm out cold. We land at LaGuardia and jump in a cab back to the city. It's a short thirty-minute ride to the West Side. It's almost 8:00 p.m. by the time we get back to my apartment.

SEAL throws a banana at me and says, "Fuel up." I have only eaten airport food all day and I'm starving. I'd love to order in Josie's, the local health food restaurant, but that's not on SEAL's menu. His specials tonight are tossed bananas and running miles.

"Let's knock these three little miles out," he says. "Six in the a.m. and three miles at night," he repeats. "We need to build this foundation."

Maybe I'm calculating wrong but we did 8.3 miles this a.m. If we round up, we are done for the day.

I'm not 100 percent sure why SEAL agreed to come "work" with me. As eager as I was to shake up my life, I bet in some way he was equally curious to see how I lived. To learn. To get some ideas about business, travel, family, and life after the military. I'm not really sure. It's too early in our relationship, but I make a mental note to ask him down the road.

Winter in NYC can be very cold, and tonight the big CNN video screen that's displayed across from my apartment says seventeen degrees. SEAL puts on the same outfit he has had on for the past five runs. I mean the exact same outfit. How did all his shit dry?

I go into my room and layer up in long-sleeve running shirts. I also grab two hats and throw them on. It's a universally accepted fact that you lose a lot of warmth through your head. If you keep your head warm in the severe cold, you will have won half the battle of keeping your body warm. I usually always prefer to run in shorts (regardless of the temperature), but tonight I choose to put on a thin thermal legging because it's so damn cold.

During the ride down the thirty-seven flights on the elevator, SEAL doesn't even look at me. It's like he's infuriated with me. Actually, he looks like he is mad at something way bigger than just me. Is he mad at the world?

"Let's get the fuck out of here," he says as the elevator opens. "Fuck it. Let's do six," SEAL says as we leave. I don't even question it 'cause he looks so mad.

We run six miles in Central Park. Usually I run the loop of Central Park in a clockwise direction, but tonight he wants to run it in the opposite direction. He tells me we hit way more hills going this way. Not sure I really get that. To me it sounds like a word problem I had in eighth-grade math, but there's no time to discuss. Off we go.

SEAL does not look at his watch once during the run,

and when we finish he hits the stop button on his GPS. I hear it beep indicating the run is done and logged. "We did those in nines," he says. He then looks down at his watch...exactly fifty-four minutes. It's like he is a human GPS.

"SEAL, how the *fuck* did you know we were running nines without checking your watch?"

"Instincts. You need to feel the pace."

This guy is like the Obi-Wan Kenobi of running!

Twenty minutes later...

It's about 10:00 p.m. and I'm starting to think about sleep. I'm usually not hungry after I work out and tonight is no different. I guzzle a glass of water and wash up. Sara is reading *People* magazine in the living room.

Ten minutes later...

I walk to SEAL's room to say good night and see if he needs anything. Our relationship is still in the infancy stages, and I want to make sure he feels welcome. I lightly knock on his door three times and then peek my head in. He's sitting upright in his bed like he knew I was going to come in.

"Hey, man," I say. "You cool?"

"You know what, Jesse?" SEAL says. "No, I'm not cool. I'm sick of this shit." SEAL pounds his fist on the bed. "You're too pretty, man. Too cute. Fuck you."

What?

"Go grab a chair. The most uncomfortable chair you can find."

I have no idea what he's talking about, but I go and get a wooden chair, one with no armrests, out of my home office and return to his room.

"This?"

"This is perfect!" SEAL says. "Sit down."

I sit in the chair.

"Now go grab a fucking blanket," he says.

"Wait. What?"

He doesn't really think I'm going to sleep in A CHAIR?

"You got to get out of your comfort zone, Jesse," he says. "Enough of this comfy shit. Fuck this Park Avenue bullshit." He repeats himself under his breath: "Fucking Park Avenue bullshit."

But we live on Central Park West...

So I grab a blanket and try to get comfortable sitting in the chair. Every time I try to stretch out to get into more of a reclined/bed position, I slide down off the chair. Then Sara walks in.

"Hey, honey! Umm...what are you doing?"

"Sweetie, SEAL says I need to get out of my comfort zone. He wants me to sleep in this chair. It must be a mental thing." I'm trying to spin this as positively as I can. It's almost like I'm trying to convince myself that this is a great idea.

"Jess, you're a forty-two-year-old father. Please go and get into your bed."

My wife knows what I signed up for, but she slightly rolls her eyes, a judgmental expression that's somewhat neutralized by her smile. Sara also knows I'm going to make every

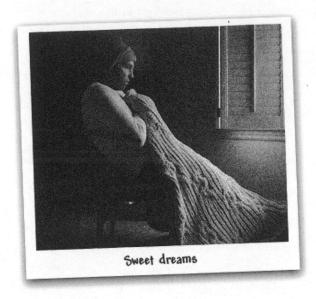

Sweet dreams

attempt to complete any and all of SEAL's challenges. But she didn't think I'd be told to sleep in a chair.

The blanket isn't helping, and the chair squeaks every time I shift positions. My wife shakes her head, turns, and walks back to the bedroom to our comfy bazillion-thread-count-sheet bed (my wife likes nice sheets).

It's midnight. Lights out.

> **Workout totals: 14.3 miles (8.3 miles in the morning and 6 miles at night)**

Sara's First Sighting

*I don't do shit for applauses. I don't do shit for
fanfare. I do shit for me.*
—SEAL

The first time Sara saw SEAL was before he moved in with
us, but after I flew to the West Coast to offer my invitation.
I'd told my wife I wanted to run the Badwater race—it's
a grueling 135-mile ultra-marathon through the Mojave
Desert's Death Valley in 130-degree heat (and that's in the
shade). Sara thought that was the dumbest thing she ever
heard and insisted I first go watch the race to see what it was
all about before I entered it myself. And like a good husband,
I agreed. And because of the extreme nature of the race and
inherent danger, she decided that she ought to come too. You
know, for a second opinion.

I'd always wanted to complete the Badwater race. It is
considered the toughest footrace on Earth, and rightfully so.
135 miles. 130-degree heat. Plus, the last thirteen miles of
the race are a straight ascent up Mount Whitney. I also knew
SEAL was running in it.

I just felt like this race was *the* race to do for my life
résumé. It was the ultimate physical and mental challenge,
and I wanted to take the test. I guess I also wanted to be able
to look other runners in the face and say, "I completed Badwater." Like I said earlier, I want to get better.

So that summer for our family "vacation," we flew across

the country in July to watch the race. Since there are no
direct flights (or any flights, for that matter) into Death Valley,
we had to fly into Las Vegas, rent a car, and drive a few hours
to the desert. The ride to Death Valley is long and boring,
straight through the desert. Not a great way to spend your
vacation if you're Sara (but I was psyched to watch the race).
We got there just after the final wave of runners started the
race. We drove out about twenty miles past the start to cheer
on the competitors.

Any description I could offer here wouldn't do justice to
how hot it was. As we arrived, the thermometer in the car
showed the outside temp to be 128 degrees. It was so hot
that at first Sara wouldn't even get out of the car. We parked
at the thirty-mile mark and watched the racers pass with the
air conditioner inside blasting.

Now, I'm not sure if you have ever seen an ultra-marathon
before, but the competitors are an interesting breed of
humans. As Sara said, "It's like they put ninety people from
an insane asylum onto a Greyhound bus, drove them out
to the desert, blew a whistle, and said run for two days."
She wasn't far off. Most of the runners looked like a cross
between scrawny science teachers and confused goat herd-
ers. As we cheered on the runners, they enjoyed our support
by thanking us and giving us high-fives. Some even engaged
in light conversation. Sara could not believe the group. She
anticipated super-fit athletes, not folks who looked like mad
scientists in running shorts.

But then, over the horizon, she saw what she thought was
a mirage coming toward us. It was like the music from *Char-
iots of Fire* started playing in Death Valley as he approached.

The guy was a machine. He stared straight ahead like there was nothing in his path and ran. His muscles were like a locomotive train. As he passed us, Sara jumped up and down and yelled, "GO! GO! GO!" Although there wasn't another human within a mile of us or him, he didn't even react. No "thank you"...no smile...no anything.

"Holy shit," she exclaimed. "What the hell was that?"

Several months later "that" moved into our house.

DAY 4

Fitness Test

I don't think about yesterday. I think about today
and getting better.
—SEAL

New York City
25°
0530

I've been in and out of sleep all night but officially wake up
in the chair at 5:30 a.m. I've never been more happy to be
up at 5:30 a.m. in my life. My neck is *KILLING* me. I have
an L-shaped back and my knees are locked. I think I got
two hours of sleep...MAX. SEAL meets me in the den at
0545. He looks like he's already showered, had coffee, and
read the morning paper. Maybe he has. He doesn't say a
word about the chair. Nothing.

Now that we are three days into his stay and have "built
a foundation," SEAL decides he wants to test where I'm at...

physically. We "agreed" last night to an 0600 start time for our "fit test." Agreed means he told me when we're waking up.

Before SEAL got here, I had no idea how to convert military time into regular human time (the time the rest of the world operates on). But now I'm completely fluent in the conversion. So, at 0545 we head down to the gym for our test.

Before we get started, SEAL takes his shirt off. He looks at himself in the gym mirror. It's almost like he is doing it in slow motion. Checking to see if he added more definition to his Hulk-like body overnight. I apologize and explain that he has to keep his clothing on in the building gym, that those are the rules . . . that other residents will be coming down soon.

He acts like I'm taking a toy away from him and telling him to brush his teeth, like it's my rule. Like I'm the stuffy one.

"That's the dumbest shit ever," he says. "This is a gym. Gyms have mirrors."

"I know but that's the rules."

"Well, whoever made that rule is an asshole."

He reluctantly keeps his shirt on, and we walk over to the pull-up bar for what he has coined "nickels and dimes." We do five pull-ups (nickels) and then ten push-ups (dimes) "every minute on the minute."

We start every time the second hand is on the 12. If we finish in forty seconds, we then have twenty seconds of rest. We do this for ten minutes (fifty pull-ups and a hundred push-ups). However, by the time we get to four minutes, I have to drop my pull-up count to three. I can't keep up. I'm a runner, but this is a totally different skill set. I assume most forty-three-year-old men aren't doing eight pull-ups, let alone fifty.

SEAL doesn't say anything. He just pulls out his tiny journal and scribbles in it.

I'm already incredibly sore and struggling. Pull-ups are not my thing. Plus I'm still sore from the pull-ups three days ago.

SEAL says, "Okay, now we get started."

"What?"

We head over to the treadmill. SEAL hands me two twenty-pound dumbbells and sets the controls. Incline: 8. Speed: 4.0. He pushes the start button. I do this for eight minutes. It's like a brisk walk up a moderate-size hill carrying a couple of suitcases. Then, every minute thereafter, SEAL increases the incline by 1. By incline 10 it feels like I'm walking up a steep hill carrying two camp trucks; by 15, I'm climbing the side of a *mountain* holding two minivans! When I'm done, my shoulder blades feel like they're on fire. My thighs are jacked up. My lungs are so expanded it feels like they're going to burst my rib cage.

SEAL pulls out his tiny journal and marks it as such.

In fact, I tell him to jot it down in bold: MISERABLE.

We head over to the box jump. It's twenty-four inches high. He times me on how long it takes me to do fifty: 1 minute, 57 seconds.

SEAL pulls out his tiny journal and marks it as such.

Then we go outside and run six miles. It takes me an hour. I'm miserable. *Miserable.*

SEAL pulls out his tiny journal and marks it as such.

What's amazing is that SEAL not only does almost every

single workout with me, *but* he also does his own personal workouts on top of this. It was like the workouts we're doing that are knocking me out are not nearly enough for him. My workouts are like his jumping jacks for a warm-up.

We have only been together for a few days and I never really see SEAL lifting weights, but the guy is always doing push-ups. It's like push-ups are his hobby or more like it's his job. Or better yet, it's his hobby *and* his job. Anytime I go into the kitchen I see him doing push-ups in his room or in the hallway. He'll be in position, pushing up and down. And completely out of nowhere the guy will just drop and give himself twenty—at work, in the lobby, in the restroom. Anywhere and everywhere. It's not normal.

Today, for example, when the doorman came to the apartment to drop off some packages that were delivered, SEAL answered the door and welcomed him in. As the doorman was placing the package by the wall, he tried to engage SEAL in conversation.

"You good?" the doorman asks.

Rather than answer and continue a normal conversation, SEAL drops to the floor and starts doing rapid-fire push-ups.

"Hey, man, just leave that shit by the wall. Appreciate it," he says as he goes up and down...up and down...up and down.

> Workout totals: 6 miles, 15-minute treadmill test, 50 box jumps, 36 pull-ups, and 100 push-ups

DAY 5

Escape Vehicle

It doesn't have to be fun. It has to be effective.
—SEAL

New York City
20°
0800

I'm on the couch reading the *New York Post*. The door to the apartment opens. It's SEAL. He's back from doing an errand.

"This is fucking amazing."

SEAL is holding a fifty-pound camouflage backpack and four oars.

"What's that for?" I set down the paper and sit up a little straighter on the couch.

"It's your escape vehicle out of Manhattan," he says. "In this backpack is an inflatable raft that carries a maximum load of 450 pounds. Pull this cord and it inflates instantly." He shows me the cord. "You, Sara, and Lazer can all fit in it comfortably and paddle to Jersey."

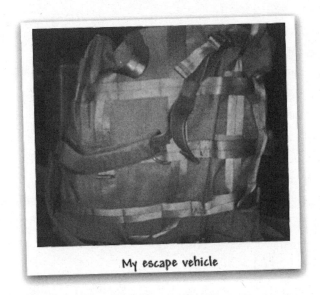

My escape vehicle

"Brilliant!" I say.

"Man, this shit is so badass," he says. "It's low to the water and impossible to see at night. It has an attachable motor. If you time your escape right, you can get out of Dodge undetected. POOF!"

This is the most animated I've seen SEAL since he got here.

"But why would we want to escape?" I ask.

"In case some 9/11 shit happens again. There's only one way out—the river. The city shuts down all bridges and tunnels and access points. How the fuck else do you plan to get out? What's the plan?"

"Plan? I don't have a plan."

"Well you do now. You're gonna row row row your boat the fuck out of here."

Makes sense to me.

As SEAL and I are admiring the fifty-pound backpack and the four oars, Sara walks in the front door.

My wife looks down at the backpack and then up at us. She is a bit confused.

"Sweetie, SEAL got us a backpack that turns into an inflatable raft in case we need to get out of the city," I say.

"An inflatable raft? We live on the thirty-seventh floor in an apartment in Manhattan."

"Yeah, SEAL said the bridges and tunnels get shut down during an emergency. It's protocol. A raft is the only way out. We just bring it to the Hudson River and inflate it. Then we paddle to New Jersey."

"Okay, love." She sets the mail down on the kitchen counter.

"That's it? Just 'okay, love'? Any thoughts?"

"Well, just so I understand. I'm supposed to grab my son, strap a fifty-pound pack on my shoulders, carry four oars, walk a mile to the river, inflate this survival raft, and then paddle to New Jersey... in the middle of a national emergency?"

There is dead silence in the room.

Then... more dead silence.

Sara chimes in and says, "I'm not even sure I could lift this thing."

"Nah, you'll be fine," SEAL says as he grabs the backpack and puts it on Sara's back.

She falls straight over backward.

I think to myself, she has a point.

Finally SEAL interjects. I can tell he is about to lose it and has been holding in his words. But now he can't hold them in any longer. "Sara, don't EVER underestimate the power of adrenaline," he says.

So we put the backpack behind the bar.

Four hours later...

"Come on, we're going to do the one hundred workout."

SEAL explains the routine, and I realize that he needs help with his math...it's really the *five hundred* workout.

We jump on the elevator and head down to the gym. There are already three other people working out when we get there. While the gym is fully operational and is loaded with equipment, it's rare that more than a handful of residents are ever there working out at the same time.

There's a guy with blond hair doing what looks like a serious core workout.

SEAL looks at the guy and then back at me.

"What the fuck is Billy Idol doing here?" SEAL asks.

"That's Sting," I whisper. "He lives in the building."

We do a hundred dumbbell bench presses (2X), no rest, and I start with thirty-pound weights but end with twenty-pounders. Total: 200.

100 lateral pull-downs (2X). 75 pounds. Total: 200
100 shoulder presses (seated). Total: 100

Like I said, that's five hundred, not one hundred.

Extra credit: 2X light triceps pull-downs and 2X curls

It's time to leave. We make our way out of the gym.

"Well, that didn't look fun," Sting says.

7:00 p.m.

It's Saturday night and most of the people I know are watching college football. Not us, because apparently SEAL does have a friend—someone he met in my gym yesterday. They must have become close because the guy lets SEAL borrow his fifty-pound weight vest. SEAL hands it to me.

"Put it on."

I grab it and put one arm in at a time. I throw the vest over my shoulders and strap it on. My immediate reaction is *This is heavy*. Like really heavy. It's like having a big suitcase on your back.

We do fifteen sets of ten push-ups, with thirty seconds of rest between sets.

Total: 150.

It takes me twenty-two minutes.

It takes SEAL fifteen minutes.

"This is no punk," SEAL says.

And it's not. It's so hard that even SEAL can't go straight to ten without dropping to his knees after the sixth set. Yet all he keeps saying is: "This is great."

This is not great. This is brutally hard.

I found out SEAL once entered a race where you could either run for twenty-four or forty-eight hours. Shocker: SEAL signed up for the forty-eight-hour one. At around the twenty-three-hour mark, he'd run approximately 130 miles, but he'd also torn his quad. He asked the race officials if they could just clock him out at twenty-four hours. When he was told they couldn't do that, he said, "ROGER THAT," asked for a roll of tape, and wrapped his quad. He walked (limped) on a torn quad for the last twenty-four hours to finish the race and complete the entire forty-eight hours.

"When you think you're done, you're only at forty percent of what your body is capable of doing. That's just the limit that we put on ourselves."

Workout totals: 500 workout (bench presses, lat pull-downs, shoulder presses) and 150 push-ups

Señoras de la Limieza

I don't need new friends. I like to keep my
shit lean and tight.
—SEAL

We have two cleaning ladies who come to the apartment twice a week. They don't speak a lick of English, and I don't speak a lick of Spanish. So I have to use props and diagrams to communicate. If I want them to vacuum, I go get a magazine and show them a picture of a vacuum. If I want them to clean the windows, I show them a photo of Windex and point to the glass.

I keep a stash of *Us Weekly* around just for communication purposes. I'm always pointing to stuff and showing them a picture of what I need them to do. It's kind of like a combination of American Sign Language and charades. It can get challenging.

But when SEAL came into their world, there was no way I could explain him to them. I mean, what do I do? Show them a picture of Russell Crowe in *Gladiator*? Or Stallone's *Rambo*? But as I've come to learn, some things don't need to be communicated. These women were immediately obsessed with him. I mean, SEAL is a nice-looking man. Have I mentioned that? And he walks around without a shirt a lot. *A lot!* In fact, I'm starting to notice that Sara's friends are coming over lately for no reason. I guess they want to just look at SEAL.

Since he's moved in, the cleaning gals seem to be spending an extra hour or two cleaning. They also seem to be spending a lot time in his room despite the fact the guy is spotless. His room doesn't need cleaning—*ever*! Military corners, you could bounce a quarter off the bed after he makes it, all his gear is stowed. I mean, the bedroom looks like it's right out of a boot camp. But the ladies are always in there when SEAL's around, talking to each other in Spanish and giggling.

In the other direction, SEAL doesn't even acknowledge them. He's not exactly rude to them, it's more like a silent assessment—and he doesn't trust them.

Yesterday he ordered something that was FedExed to the apartment and one of the cleaning ladies accepted the package, he freaked out—not to them, but to me.

"It's a breach of security," he said.

Breach of security?

"The integrity of the delivery was compromised."

He went on to lecture me about my naiveté when it comes to insubordination of the people who work for me. The only thing he ever said about anyone was they should be fired. SEAL didn't think anyone who worked for the Itzlers cared enough or did their job like they should. He was really mad or suspicious of everyone he came into contact with except for Sara, Lazer, and me. According to SEAL, if my driver, Smith, was a minute late, it was because he didn't study the routes correctly. If there was traffic, Smith should have anticipated the accident.

In looking back on it now, I'm not sure SEAL was wrong. He was taught that if you have a job to do, you do it with 120 percent effort. I have been operating under the assumption that if someone that works for me does something 80 percent of the way I would do it, that's enough. SEAL is teaching me that we can all do so much more.

DAY 6

That Damn Finger

It's really not that complicated.
—SEAL

New York City
29°
0400

It's 4:00 a.m. I hear some banging and mumbling in the living room. Banging…mumbling…banging…mumbling. Although I am half asleep, I decide to check it out.

When I get to the living room, SEAL is on the couch holding the remote control. Well, holding is not really an appropriate description. He is slamming the remote control against the armrest of the couch as if that may turn the TV on.

"This motherfucker," he mumbles, "is too complicated. Too many buttons. It's making me fucking nuts."

SEAL looks like he may implode. His eyebrows are arched and he looks like he could attack…anything. Right now, he is attacking the remote but since I'm the closest human, I'm alarmed.

So, I immediately grab the remote and hit POWER then switch the command to CABLE 1. I put on ESPN and hand SEAL the remote.

"Just use the channel and volume controls for now. No need to even shut it off. I will shut off the TV in the morning."

SEAL's eyebrows contort back to normal as he watches some football highlights.

I go back to bed.

0600.

I hear my bedroom door slowly open. There's no nice way to put this, but it's a bit unnerving because my wife is in bed next to me and I can sense someone else in the room with us. I feel a tap.

I half open my eyes and imagine I see a long black finger on my shoulder. I roll over. My wife is sound asleep. Plus, the finger I'm imagining doesn't look anything like her finger.

I ignore the finger. I must be dreaming.

Ten seconds later, I feel another tap on my shoulder. I'm hoping it's my wife, but this finger does not belong to her. The finger keeps tapping me. In the other hand, is a remote.

I ignore it again.

Twenty seconds later, I feel hot breath whispering into my ear in a monotone voice. I guess the loud-intentional-noises-in-the-hallway trick wasn't working for him.

"Get up, motherfucker," SEAL says.

I get up. Fast. Sara remains motionless and oblivious next to me.

SEAL tells me we'll run another six miles in Central Park this a.m. That this is our last "primer." Then we start.

Start? I thought we started days ago.

I go into the living room and shut the TV off.

Central Park is where most of our training occurs. Park Drive is a 6.1-mile loop in the heart of Manhattan. Back in the 1970s, before they routed the race through the five boroughs, the New York City Marathon was held in Central Park. The marathoners ran around the loop four times plus. I've run the course hundreds of times since I moved to Manhattan, as it serves as a perfect training ground with its rolling hills, few cars at this time of the morning (which probably disappoints SEAL), and other runners and bikers to interact with.

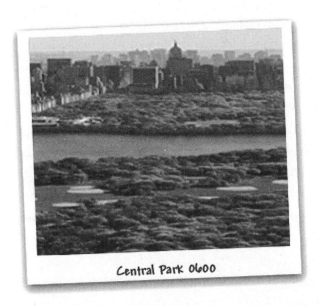

Central Park 0600

It's chilly today with the wind, but only until we start running. Our breath comes out in puffs of white. That's all that comes out of SEAL. He doesn't make a sound. He runs like a submarine. Silent. Deadly. The thought reminds me of a fart joke I heard in the fifth grade.

We do the first three miles at a ten-minute pace. Then the next two at an eight-minute pace. And the final mile is seven minutes. When we get home my son is still asleep. So is my wife. She doesn't even know there was a finger tapping me in bed earlier.

The past two days when we came home from our morning runs I have been drenched in sweat. *Soaked.* My routine has been simple: I shower, grab a bowl of fruit and some bananas, then go to work.

I eat only fruit until noon. That's been my thing since I read *Fit for Life* by Harvey Diamond in 1992. For over twenty-five years, just fruit till noon.

Harvey is another of the "interesting people" that I cold-called to be my friend. His story is fascinating. Harvey was exposed to Agent Orange, perhaps the most toxic molecule ever synthesized by man, during the Vietnam War. Agent Orange has been linked to various cancers, lymphomas, and multiple chronic diseases.

As far as I know, Harvey is the only American soldier who was exposed to the deadly chemical and is still alive. He credits it to a philosophy and lifestyle called "natural hygiene," and he lays out the road map in *Fit for Life*. I read the book three times, and it completely changed my life.

So one day I decided to call Harvey and introduce

myself. No different from SEAL. I tracked down his number, picked up the phone, and got him on the line. He checked the "yes" box to being my friend and we have been great friends since.

He's another character in my life that my wife tolerates. Every time we talk, he ends the call with "Fruit till noon, brother." One of the main underlying philosophies in his book is that we use more energy for digestion than all other bodily functions combined. That's why we are usually tired after a big meal. That said, the average American will eat seventy tons of food in their lifetime. Imagine how hard the body has to work to process and break down all of that food. The more efficiently we can digest all this food and the less stress we put on the digestive process, the more energy we will have for everything else.

According to *Fit for Life*, fruit is the perfect food because on top of being sweet and delicious, it's super-easy to digest. In fact, it is the only food that bypasses the stomach and is digested in the small intestines. It unleashes all its nutrients and goodness without using much, if any, energy, which frees up your energy for other things. As long as you eat fruit on an empty stomach, you can reap amazing benefits.

According to Diamond, you don't have to look beyond the animal kingdom to see evidence of this. The strongest animals in the world thrive on a fruit- and plant-based diet. Silverback gorillas, for example, are thirty times as strong as man and three times our size. Their DNA is 99 percent similar to that of humans, and they are our closest living relatives next to chimps. How are they so strong? Oh yeah, their diet is made up mostly of fruit and leaves. The silverback gorilla doesn't eat turkey sandwiches, chips, and McDonald's. Makes sense to me.

After reading the book in 1992, I decided to try the concept out for myself. I religiously stuck to a fruit-only diet until noon every day for ten days. After noon I generally kept it pretty clean—no fried foods, no dairy, no meats, but I didn't waver from the fruit *only* in the a.m. I had an enormous amount of energy during that span and very "efficient" digestion. I felt so good that the ten-day trial period turned into twenty-plus years of following this routine. It doesn't matter if I'm running a full marathon in the morning; I still stick to this program. Fruit till noon!

1:00 p.m.

Forty-five minutes after I get to the office this morning, SEAL arrives.

I'm back sitting in front of my computer when he gets there. I ordered in a salmon platter and some veggie dumplings from Josie's. I ate them like a wrestler right after his weigh-in. It's been about an hour since I had lunch. Zico's marketing team has presented some new packaging, and we are reviewing the options. SEAL sits in a chair in my office, motionless. That is, until he jumps out of the chair, unprompted.

"Burpee test, motherfucker," he barks.

"I'm sorry, what?"

"Burpee test, motherfucker. Why do I have to keep repeating myself?"

"I just didn't know what you meant."

"Dude, you know what a fucking burpee is, right?" He's not really asking but telling me.

"Yeah, I know what a burpee is."

"And you know what a motherfuckin' test is, right?"

"Yes. I know what a test is."

"Well then, motherfucker, this is a burpee test."

SEAL tells me he wants to time how long it takes me to do a hundred burpees. "It's a fitness test," he says, and makes sure to emphasize these are burpees with push-ups. He explains that anything under ten minutes is solid, under eleven minutes is acceptable, and he finds over thirteen minutes is unacceptable.

"In fact, if you don't go under thirteen minutes, we are doing them again," he says.

Well, I'm not really good at burpees, and I find doing one set of fifteen to be a friggin' pain.

SEAL takes off his watch and presses the start button.

BEEP!

"Wait, I have to change into something."

"Clock's already started, bitch."

I immediately drop to the floor in a plank position, do a push-up, kick my knees to my chest, and jump up into a jumping jack. One.

I get to ten in fifty-five seconds. I'm on pace. Problem is, I'm already starting to sweat, and I'm in my work clothes. I'm in my work clothes *because* . . . I'm at work. Plus, I need to look presentable for my meetings today. I don't want to get them all sweaty.

So, I use or waste, however you want to look at it, the next ten precious seconds taking my shirt off and then my shoes and socks. And finally my pants. I'm now in my boxers in my office. Eleven, twelve, thirteen...I keep going.

The clock is ticking and I'm at fifty at 5:30. I'm slowing down, but I'm still on pace for "acceptable." I can feel sweat on my face and rolling down the center of my back.

The door opens.

But I only see the back of her head before the blond hair quickly exits.

It's Jennifer Kish, my right-hand person at the office. She's gone before I can explain. I want to yell "burpee test, motherfucker" but the door is already closed behind her. I wonder what she's thinking.

I keep going.

When I get to sixty, I start breaking down the remaining forty burpees into sets of ten. Ten burpees and then a ten- to fifteen-second rest.

Eleven minutes, forty-five seconds. Done.

I grab an old T-shirt I happen to have lying around and wipe myself off. I'm soaked. It takes about twenty minutes for me to stop sweating, and my thighs feel like they are *broken*. I throw the soaking-wet T-shirt into the garbage can by my desk and put on my work clothes.

Soon enough I'm back at my computer looking at the color options on the packaging. My legs tremble and shake under my desk. Work resumes and a slight smile comes over my face as I think, *Burpee test, bitch!*

I work for nine hours straight.

2200

I walk home from work at 10:00 p.m. with SEAL. It's been a long day. We've been working on Zico all day with the design people, and I'm wiped out. While we were able to be additive with the new packaging, a big part of our role is generating sizzle for the brand. Every day we ask ourselves: How do we generate buzz and excitement around our products? But generating the buzz today took a lot out of me. I just want to turn on the television. Maybe watch the fourth quarter of the Knicks game and veg out. I lie down on the couch and look for the remote. SEAL has been with me all day at the office, and he's seen how intense it's been. The only real time I was alone today was when I went to the bathroom. It might have been the best five minutes of my day. I'm beat, so I'm not going to say anything about working out if he doesn't, plus we have already run six miles and done one hundred burpees. I grab the remote and flip on the television.

SEAL doesn't watch much TV. I feel like he just watches me watch TV. It's very uncomfortable. And it makes me not want to watch TV.

"You a Knicks fan?" he asks.

"All my life," I say.

"You ever go to the games?"

"I do," I say. I've had season tickets for years. "I even wrote their theme song back in the day."

"A song?"

"Rap song, theme song sort of like an anthem," I say, then

sing a little: "*Go New York, Go New York, Go...* You ever hear of it?"

"That's it?"

"That's what?"

"That's the whole song?"

"No. That's only the chorus, there's a whole verse and then you repeat the chorus, you know?"

"Doesn't seem that complicated."

"I'm not sure if it's complicated or if it's simple, but I do know that it worked," I respond.

I was a twenty-three-year-old recording artist signed to a small independent record label called Delicious Vinyl when I wrote "Go New York Go" in 1993. I somehow convinced the Knicks brass they needed a new theme song and that we could get Spike Lee and other celebs in a video around the song if we did it correctly. They gave me a shot. "Go New York Go" became the Knicks' anthem and the number-one most requested song on New York radio during the 1993–1994 NBA playoffs. The lyrics were licensed by Budweiser, Foot Locker, and other major brands. I felt like I had finally *arrived*. I was *big time*.

Well, not really big time. The Knicks paid me $4,000 to write the song. After I paid the studio, engineer, producer, and musicians, I think I netted about $300, and a net worth of $300 isn't really big time. But to me it was. Any success I have ever had in my life usually occurred when I was *not* chasing the money but was doing things out of passion. And as far as music, I was never in it for the money.

But it's not like I just woke up one day and said I want to write and record a hip-hop theme song for the New York Knicks. It started much earlier than that.

After graduation from American University, my plan A was to get a record deal and to be on MTV. That's it. There was no plan B. There was no financial goal. I just wanted to be on MTV.

Getting a record deal is one of the hardest things you can ever do. The odds of even getting a meeting with the right person are very low, and the odds of getting signed—well, those are virtually astronomical. If you don't have a powerful lawyer or know someone, then the astronomical odds become...ridiculously astronomical. I didn't have either.

In 1988, a show on MTV called *Yo! MTV Raps* debuted. The program was like the Jackie Robinson of rap TV—it broke all sorts of barriers and injected rap into mainstream culture. Still, by 1990, you could count the number of white hip-hop artists who were receiving any kind of acceptance in the larger community on one of Ice Cube's hands. The Beastie Boys were at the top of the list along with 3rd Bass. Maybe it was naiveté or pure determination—probably both—but despite the enormous odds facing me, I knew what I was going to do. I was going to be on *Yo! MTV Raps*.

A few weeks after "Pomp and Circumstance" played at my graduation ceremony, I got a phone call from a fraternity brother who had moved to LA to be a production assistant on a movie called *The Bonfire of the Vanities*. As he got settled in California, he invited me out to LA to check out the movie set (uh-hemm...and the girls).

I had never been to Cali, so I hopped on a plane and headed west.

At the time, there was a hot new independent label called Delicious Vinyl located off Sunset Boulevard. Delicious was an ultra-hip recording outfit with two of the hottest artists on pop radio: Tone-Loc and Young MC. Loc's song "Wild Thing" was the number-one-selling single in the country, and Young's "Bust a Move" was blowing up the charts. If I could write my own script, this would be the perfect label for me. Fun. Irreverent. Successful. Different. I had to meet the owners.

The guy who was the head of Delicious was named Mike Ross. In the music business, creating and distributing a song usually works like this: There's the artist who is signed by a label. Once that deal is done, either the artist has a particular producer they always work with to create and record the songs (Michael Jackson, for example, was always produced by Quincy Jones), or the label hires a producer to work with the artist. That is, of course, unless the artist does it all himself. Mike Ross was one of those rare label owners who also produced the music his label released. Along with his partner, Matt Dike, Ross was one of the most dynamic rap producers in the business.

I had read that Mike was a big fan of a Brooklyn-born rapper named Dana Dane. A big fan. As it turns out, Dana Dane recorded at Hurby "Luv Bug" Azor's studio (the same studio I recorded at), and one night while I was at the studio, I saw an advance copy of Dana's album lying on the mix board. I decided to "borrow" it while nobody was looking. Couldn't hurt. It was his second album and highly anticipated in the music community. I brought the cassette with me to LA. Nobody outside of Dana's inner clique had even heard it yet.

After only two days in LA, I decided to cold-call Mike Ross at Delicious Vinyl. "Why not?" I thought. If I was going to take a shot, I might as well take one from outside the arc. I literally got his office number out of the phone book and called the main line. I didn't have a game plan other than try to get a meeting with Mike:

"Delicious Vinyl, may I help you?" the receptionist said.

"Mike Ross, please."

"Sure, please hold."

Forty-five seconds later...

"This is Dina, Mike Ross's assistant. Can I help you?"

"Mike, please."

"Mike's not in. Who's calling?"

"Jesse."

"Jesse who?"

"Jesse. I'm a friend of Dana Dane's. Dana wanted me to drop off his new cassette for Mike while I'm in town. I'm leaving tomorrow. He said it's urgent. Mike knows about it."

"Please hold."

I covered the receiver with my hand and whispered to my friend Jon. "I'm on hold."

Maybe it was my thick Long Island accent disconnecting with her Cali vibe or maybe it was the universe wanting me to get in that door, but thirty seconds later she comes back:

"So you're Dana Dane?"

Obviously I don't look like Dana (he's African American and I'm white...he has a gold front tooth and I don't...etc.). I guess I could have cleared up the misunderstanding right then and there, *but*...when your foot is half in the door, you don't pull it out. So, without pausing, I say...

"Yes! I'm Dana."

"Okay, hold on."

One minute later...

"Dana, Mike is excited to meet you. Can you come in today around 2:00 p.m.?"

"Yes, ma'am. I'll be there."

Game on, motherfucker!

At precisely two o'clock I show up at the Delicious Vinyl offices. I'm twenty-one years old. I walk up the stairs to the second floor, where the buzzer to announce yourself is located. I push the button for entry. A very sexy receptionist voice chimes in through the speaker box:

"Who is it?"

"Oh, it's Dana Dane here to see Mike Ross please," I respond.

Ten seconds later...

BUZZZZZZ.

I'm in!

Mike Ross's assistant leads me to his office and sits me down right on the chair across from Mike's big-ass executive desk. "Mike will be back in five minutes, Dana," she tells me, right before she offers me some water.

She closes the door behind her and there I am. Just me...sitting in Mike's big, cool, unlit office. There are gold records hanging on the walls, different album covers, photos, and really cool graffiti. A patchouli candle is burning on his desk. The office is amazing. I start to read the credits on Tone-Loc's platinum album hanging on the wall and check out some of the awards on Mike's desk. Then the door opens and Mike Ross appeared. He is baffled.

"Who are you?" he said.

"What's up, Mike? I'm Jesse. I work with Dana. He's running a little late."

"Late?

"Yeah, he's maybe like twenty minutes behind."

"How do you know Dana?"

(I'd never met Dana.)

"I record with him at the same studio. My producer is part of his production crew called Idolmakers, and I did a few songs for him too."

"You sing?"

"No. I actually rap."

"You rap? With Dana?"

I figured I would continue to confuse him as it has worked thus far...

"Yeah. Well, not with him directly, but I'm part of a group signed to Virgin. But Dana thinks I should do a solo thing."

"Virgin? Do you have any songs with you?"

"Yeah! I do. Can I pop this cassette in while we wait?"

"Sure."

I handed Mike a copy of my three-song demo, and "College Girls" comes on first.

Anywhere I go a fly girl will please me
East to west college girls are easy.

He listens for thirty seconds and stops the tape.

"This is fucking amazing."

"Man, thanks, brother. I think it's a hit!"

"Who is your lawyer?"

"Excuse me?"

"Who is your lawyer?" he asks again.

And just like that—just like that!!!—after two years of getting doors slammed in my face, he hit me with the four magic words every artist shopping a demo tape wants to hear: *"Who is your lawyer?"* In fact, he asked me twice!

Since I didn't have a lawyer and I didn't even know any lawyers, I told him: "Oh, my dad is."

"Your dad is an entertainment lawyer?"

At the time my dad owned a plumbing supply company, but it was the first answer that popped into my head (I'm a "get your foot in the door, figure it out later guy") so I responded with a firm "Yes." "Yep…my dad does all my stuff."

"I'm gonna have my attorney contact your dad. I want to buy this song for Loc."

"That's incredible, if Loc did this song…" Then I paused. Loc? I realized that this song was *my* ticket to a deal. Sure,

I could have sold it to Tone-Loc. "Wild Thing" had sold over 3 million units at the time, but this was the lead song on my demo. So I responded, "Actually, I really think this song is a big hit. I gotta keep this one for me. It's going on *my* album."

"That makes sense. Well, would you be willing to write for Loc then?"

And that was the *official* start of my music career.

Mike gave me the instrumentals for four songs he wanted me to write for Tone-Loc and sent me back to my friend's apartment. Two hours later, I called him on his Nokia with lyrics for all of the songs. He was at a Dodgers game and could barely hear me over the din of the stadium. But he heard enough to meet me back at his office when the game was over. There I not only signed a deal to write songs for Tone-Loc, but he signed me on the spot for my own album. (Dana later became a great friend and we still laugh about it.) Thanks, Dana!

Maybe the best part about my music career was the fact that I didn't sell that many records. As my wife likes to say, "Failure is just life's way of nudging you and letting you know you're off course." Yes, I was on MTV and got to tour the country, but the hockey-stick-curve sales trajectory wasn't there. So, I decided to "call an audible" and look for other opportunities in music. Writing theme songs for sports teams seemed like a great niche. I loved music. Loved sports. And *nobody* else was doing it. The result was "Go New York Go." I started a niche . . . sports music.

There must be an echo in here because I keep hearing SEAL say "Doesn't seem that complicated." SEAL is a lot of things, but he is not a music critic. Rather than debate this, out of my mouth comes:

"You're right. It's really not that complicated. Pretty simple actually."

"Yeah, it's simple," he says.

I start flipping the channels. I don't even find the Knicks game on the tube before SEAL suggests we take the conversation outside and get in another workout. It's 10:45 p.m. The upside is this is the first time he's actually asking questions about me. Not that I want him to, but it makes it easier to get to know someone when there's a back-and-forth. As my wife likes to remind me, "When I talk to you…please play tennis with me and hit the ball back. It's called 'communication,' and it's important to a marriage." And although I'm not looking to get married to SEAL, my wife has a valid point.

Our workout is basically the same routine as the morning, a loop around Central Park, except tonight comes with a bonus: Every half mile we do twenty-five push-ups. The other difference is that SEAL wants the pace to escalate, meaning every mile has to be slightly faster than the previous mile.

We start out at a nine-minute pace and at 4:30 into the run, we drop and do twenty-five push-ups, then we increase to an 8:50-mile pace and 4:25 into the run, we drop and do twenty-five push-ups. This continues all the way down to an 8:10 pace for the last mile.

Every time we drop to do the push-ups, blood rushes to my head and I get slightly faint. I'm breathing so hard when we do the push-ups (plus it's friggin' *brick cold* outside) that I'm slightly hyperventilating. SEAL is knocking out the push-ups like a programmed robot. Up. Down. Up. Down. Up. Down. I'm at around nine by the time he is done with his twenty-five and already standing to start running again. Every time.

> **Workout totals: 12 miles (6 miles "escalation" pace), 300 push-ups, and 100 burpees**

DAY 7

Mix Up Your Runs

If it doesn't suck, we don't do it.
—SEAL

New York City to Atlanta
36° to 75°
0530

"Your runs are too predictable," SEAL says as he stares at me stone-faced.

"Predictable?"

"Yeah, motherfucker…predictable. It's like your legs know what's coming next. It's making shit too comfy. Your body is used to your bullshit jogging routine. Gear up and meet me in five; we're doing intervals."

I throw on my gear and grab a brand-new pair of New Balance running shoes. I have been wearing New Balance for twenty years. They are the only things I run in. Once the bottoms get fairly worn out (but not all the way worn out), I replace them with a new pair. I read that having the proper cushion on your sneakers minimizes the impact on your legs when running and therefore reduces the chance of injury. I don't know if that is true or if that was created by a sneaker company, but I bought into it hook, line, and sneaker. Regardless, New Balance are part of my routine.

Five minutes later, we're on our way to Central Park for a seven-mile run. We do the first mile at a ten-minute pace to warm up, then every quarter mile after that we runasfastaswecan. After sprinting a quarter mile we slow down to a ten-minute pace again.

SEAL pushes me so hard on the quarter miles I can feel my pulse pounding in my neck. I can literally take my pulse by just counting the thumps exploding through my neck.

At the end of the run I'm gasping for air. But it's not my heart or lungs I'm worried about.

"Man, my legs are really messed up. It feels like a knife is in my calf," I complain. "Like I can cramp any second." I grab my leg and walk stiff-legged, keeping my legs totally straight like Herman Munster from *The Munsters*.

"Perfect," SEAL says. "There's only one rule in training: If it doesn't suck, we don't do it."

I probably should have broken in my new sneakers because I feel a blister forming on my right big toe. It hurts, but that pain is trumped by the pain in my calf. The blister is more like the middle child at the dinner table—not even part of the conversation. It's like I don't even pay it any mind, but I know it's there. It's like SEAL has made blisters that previously would have been big deals almost seem insignificant.

As a reward for my pain, I get to do 275 push-ups when we get home. To make matters worse, SEAL tells me we are doing them wet.

"Wet?"

"Wet!"

"What does wet mean in push-up land?"

He tells me that we don't change out of our wet, sweaty-ass clothing. We do the push-ups wet.

"Why are we doing wet push-ups?"

"'Cause that's the way I ordered them up today. That's why. I don't give a fuck how you give them to me, but I want all two seventy-five."

This guy is out of his mind.

I drop down and do my first set of ten. My body heat is dropping fast as I cool off from the run. I'm starting to get very cold. Like shivering cold. Every time my shirt touches my skin, it feels like a wet ice pack. I look at SEAL and he is warm. Lukewarm. He is just going down, up, down, up, down, up. Fifty. Down, up, down, up...sixty...Who is this motherfucker, and where did he come from?

I don't know much about SEAL's childhood, but I do know that he always wanted to be in the Special Forces. The other day while we were sitting around he mentioned that he used to play Rambo as a kid. *Not* the way I would play Rambo (with a Toys "R" Us Rambo doll), but like real Rambo.

When SEAL was fifteen or sixteen, he would go out into the deep woods alone around 11:00 p.m. and pretend he was picking off the enemy. He said he would stay out there for hours at a time training. I found the story to be very interesting and scary.

I don't know when it dawned on me, but at some point during that story I realized I had a Navy SEAL living in my house now—for every second of the day. This guy is using my toilet, he's in my fridge, he's answering my door, and he's sleeping in the room next to my kid's. He's everywhere. I mean, I knew I had a Navy SEAL living with me in *theory* because I invited him, but in practice it was slightly disconcerting.

In fact, I'm starting to realize I know very little about SEAL. Actually, I don't really know *anything* about him. It's sorta like inviting your taxi driver home to live with you and your family and having him drive you everywhere, but you know nothing about the taxi driver.

So now I'm wondering: What if I say something he doesn't like politically? What if I say something that pisses him off? What if I accidentally offend him and he gets even angrier than he already is? I mean, I did a full background check before I hired my first assistant, and she came from a nice family I already knew. SEAL is trained to eliminate the enemy if ordered and is now living with me…and I have done nothing.

Luckily, I keep these thoughts in my head.

I know I'm being a little crazy and there's probably nothing to worry about. I mean, really. But, honestly, what the fuck was I thinking? I don't even like strangers being in my house for a couple of minutes. I hate it when the cable guy comes. And yet I now have a trained hunting machine in my midst—not only my midst, but my wife's and my son's midst. He's right in the middle of our midst.

I wish there was someone I could talk to about this. I'd tell my wife, but I can't because it'll scare her. And then she'd be like, "You have to get rid of him." And I know there's no way I can get rid of him. How can you get rid of someone like him? "Oh, excuse me, Mr. SEAL, this isn't working out, so get your gear and beat it." Right?!

So instead I do the exact opposite and say stuff to my wife like, "You know, SEAL's the nicest guy…" Or "It's really amazing how someone who looks so indestructible and scary can be so cool." I have to oversell him. But I think Sara is starting to see through my ruse. Thank God, SEAL is the perfect houseguest. He's quiet, clean, and well mannered. And thank God he and Sara are getting along well.

Seven hours later….

We show up at Teterboro Airport in New Jersey at 1:30 p.m. for our flight to Atlanta, where Spanx, my wife's company, is headquartered. Today we are flying on a Marquis Jet Citation X. I love the Citation X because it is superfast but also quite roomy. It can knock off significant travel time on a flight like this.

In the late 1990s my partner at the time, Kenny Dichter, and I were guests on a private plane. From the minute we stepped on board we were in love with the convenience of flying private; comfort and ease at its very best. When we got home from the trip, we never wanted to get back on a commercial plane again. We assumed if we wanted to fly this way, there must be a heck of a lot of others who would want to as well. There has to be a market for this, we thought.

At the time, there were only three ways to fly private: One was to buy your own plane, which was impossible unless you were Mark Cuban or the Sultan of Brunei; two, buy a fraction of a jet, which comes with a very expensive five-year commitment; or, three, charter a plane, a process that has a lot of moving parts and inconsistencies. None of those options was very appealing to us, nor would they be appealing to any potential clients if we tried to start a company, which we had begun to think about.

We wanted to create something more realistic for a much larger demographic—people who wanted to fly privately a few times a year. So we came up with this idea: What if you could buy twenty-five hours a year of private flight time? It would be almost like a Starbucks card, or a prepaid gift card, to fly.

At the time NetJets was the 800-pound gorilla of fractional jet ownership. Warren Buffett owned the company. The CEO was a guy named Richard Santulli, and the president was a guy named Jim Jacobs. When we got the idea for Marquis Jet, we knew the first call we should make was to Jacobs.

A couple of years before, during the time I was still in music and connected to a lot of artists, I'd gotten a call from a friend who wanted a favor. I don't really remember why, maybe he was doing a business deal or maybe he just wanted to do something nice for someone, but he asked me if I could get tickets to a Christina Aguilera concert in Connecticut for a friend's daughter. My friend knew that I had a relationship with Christina's manager. So I called up the manager and not only did I get the guy and his daughter great seats, but I worked out having his daughter onstage as a backup singer if she wanted to (they would shut her mic off). I mean, for a teenager, this was a life-altering moment.

The next day the guy who went to the concert with his daughter called me up and said, "I don't know who you are, but I want to let you know that I owe you one in a big way. If there's anything I can ever do…"

That guy was Jim Jacobs.

So now it's a year later, and there *is* something Jim Jacobs can do for me. I call him. I think it took him five minutes just to figure out who I was: "Who is this again?" Jim asked.

"Jesse. Christina Aguilera. Not only backstage but *on*stage," I said. "Genie in a Bottle Itzler? You said if I ever needed anything to call you." It was the same shit as when I got my record deal, I confused him. Just throwing words at him. It was Harry Truman who said, "If you can't convince them, confuse them." It's a tactic I still use instinctively. It buys time.

"Oh, yeah," he said.

"Can I steal thirty minutes of your time?" I said.

We set up a meeting with Jim Jacobs and Rich Santulli a week later. Kenny and I drove to their Woodbury, New

Jersey, headquarters with our PowerPoint deck and presentation ready to start our new private jet timeshare company. We weren't exactly sure at the time what the company was, but we knew we had a great idea. We walked into the meeting and Jim and Rich were already seated in their conference room. They were suited up, and I mean Italy suited up. About twenty minutes into the meeting, Rich Santulli said, "No way am I letting two twenty-nine-year-olds use my fleet of five hundred planes. Good to meet you, guys." Then he threw us out of his office.

"I guess we need a new idea," I said to Kenny after we walked out of there. And that's when my phone rang. It was Jim.

When I started apologizing to him for wasting his time, he cut me off.

"That was amazing! Great meeting," he said.

"Great meeting?"

"Yeah, Rich doesn't give twenty minutes to anyone. I think it went great. The idea is brilliant! I think there's something here. Why don't you tweak your presentation a little bit and come back? Let me see if I can get you another meeting."

By this time, I knew a lot of athletes and entertainers and Kenny knew a lot of Wall Street guys we both felt would be interested in buying twenty-five hours of private jet time if it was available. We realized we needed a different pitch. We needed to show Santulli and Jacobs, not tell them. So we put together our own focus group.

A week later, we were back in Santulli's office with Carl

Banks from the New York Giants, the guys from Run-DMC, a top sports agent for NBA players, and a successful Wall Street guy who ran his own firm and wanted to use jets occasionally for entertaining. One by one our focus group participants explained to Rich how they would never buy a NetJets fraction, but they *would* spend 100K or 200K on a jet card every year. They discussed how they needed the flexibility of being able to choose their flights year by year. And they talked about why they or their clients would buy a card. And how if things went well, they would eventually graduate into the fractional program NetJets already offered.

Although Santulli didn't take the bait right away, we could tell he was nibbling. It would take three or four more meetings to set the hook, but eventually Santulli told us if we were willing to put up our own money to try this idea we were calling "Marquis Jet," then he'd give us a shot at it. We did and it worked. BIG TIME.

Sara and SEAL don't really say much to each other on the plane—it's only been seven days since he moved in and they haven't had much quality time with each other—but there is a mutual respect and friendship forming.

Sara acts 100 percent normal around SEAL, as if it's not strange at all having a Navy SEAL shadow me 24/7 all of a sudden. But her disposition being normal is not abnormal to me, as sometimes my wife is in her own world. I mean, she is *brilliant* but also has her blond moments. I like to say she is 50 percent Lucille Ball and 50 percent Einstein. For example, she built a highly successful global brand with just $5,000 of savings but asks me what day of the week it is often, and means it. That said, as long as she gets seven hours of sleep and has her Starbucks in hand when the sun comes up, life is good.

My wife's name is Sara Blakely, and she's the founder and inventor of Spanx. If you're a woman, you probably know what Spanx are. If you're a guy, Sara is like the Michael Jordan of women's underwear.

When I first started dating her, I didn't get it. But now, after witnessing the love for her brand firsthand, I totally do. Women go crazy for her products. Strangers are always hugging Sara and flashing her their undergarments in public. It's wild.

What I love most about Sara's story is that, growing up, she always wanted to be a lawyer, but she failed the LSATs... twice. So instead of heading to law school after college, she decided to go to Disney World and try out to be Goofy... naturally. When she arrived, she was too short for the job (minimum height is 5'8" and Sara is 5'6") so they asked her to be a chipmunk instead.

After a short stint at Disney, Sara accepted a job with an office supply company called Danka and sold fax machines door to door... for seven years. One night before heading out for a party, she didn't like the way her own butt looked in white pants. She took a pair of scissors and cut off the feet of her pantyhose to avoid panty lines and have a smoother look under her clothes. Voilà, her invention was born.

Over the course of the next two years, Sara worked on

developing her new idea after work, at night, and on the weekends. She took $5,000 she had set aside in savings to start the company. Since she had never taken a business course in her life, she operated on instinct and guts.

Instead of using her entire budget on legal fees to patent her product, Sara bought a book on patents and wrote her own patent. She used bold colors on her packaging to make her products pop off the shelves. She spent twelve hours a day in department stores promoting her products. It worked!

The name Spanks came to Sara while sitting in traffic in Atlanta. She knew that Kodak and Coca-Cola were two of the most recognized brand names in the world and that both names shared a strong "k" sound. She figured it must be good luck. She changed the "ks" to an "x" at the last minute because she had read that made-up words are easier to trademark than real words.

Sara trademarked the company online for $150 at www.uspto.com. Today Spanx has over 150 products, hundreds of employees, and is sold worldwide.

Our newly SEAL-infused family touches down in Atlanta and we start to gather our things. Needless to say, we spend a lot of time in Atlanta because Spanx is headquartered here, but I'm not ready to give up on New York just yet. The amount of time we're spending here is also increasing, so we're renovating a new house. It's exactly two miles from our current house in Atlanta. Sara wants to check on the progress of construction.

SEAL tells me we'll run there and back as we pull into the driveway. Sara teases she will drive there and she will drive back. We quickly change and head out on our run to the house to meet Sara.

It's a nice leisurely run along shaded streets lined with beautiful homes and huge trees. We're not really pounding it and I'm thinking about how pleasant everything is today. Then, just about a mile into our run, I hear something that sounds like the crack of a huge thunderbolt. I can't pinpoint where the sound is coming from or what it is, but it sounds dangerous and close. In that instant, I turn to look at SEAL. But his arms are stretched out and he's heading toward me. He looks like an eagle. There's a woman who happens to be walking her dog on the sidewalk about five feet away. Now SEAL has both of us in his wingspan and is practically lifting us off the ground as he pushes us. It's then I see a huge branch fall twenty-five feet from a tree directly above us. It hits the ground with a massive *thud* and explodes. The thing is about eighteen inches in diameter and bursts into small pieces when it hits the cement. It would have killed us.

"Let's go. Keep pace," SEAL says, and continues on.

The entire rest of the run I'm in complete awe. It was almost as if he knew the branch would fall. How did he identify what was going on so quickly, and how did he know where the branch was coming from? This was not the type of shit you learn in a manual.

When we get to the new home, I'm still half in shock.

"How was your run?" Sara asks.

I look at SEAL expecting him to say something about the branch. Instead, he says: "Good. Your husband is improving."

Good?

He doesn't mention the branch. It was like branches falling and almost hitting him in the head is a regular thing. No biggie. Not worth a mention.

2045

Sara's watching *Oprah* repeats and I'm in my go-to-sleep clothes. SEAL appears in my room to check up on me.

"How ya legs feel?" he asks.

"Terrible. They're sore and tight."

"Cool. Put your shorts and sneakers on."

"No," I say.

"Oh, yes indeed."

It's our third run of the day. I've previously done some two-a-days while training for long races or to try to get in fast shape, but three-a-days is new territory, especially at this intensity. And especially at my age. And really especially at 8:45 p.m. at night.

One and a half miles into our six-mile run, SEAL talks for the first time.

"You okay?"

"No. I don't feel well," I say as I keep pace.

"Fuck, yeah," he celebrates. "Now you're seeing what it's like to train, Jesse. I hope you enjoy this shit." He begins to laugh, which soon becomes an all-out cackle. "You look like a pile of spilt fuck," he says.

When we return, Sara is still watching *Oprah*. It's like we never even left.

> **Workout totals: 17 miles and 275 push-ups in the morning**

DAY 8

No Peeing Allowed

This isn't piss time. It's run time.
—SEAL

Atlanta to New York City
34° to 18°
0800

After a super-early flight from Atlanta, we land back in Teterboro. The flight time to Teterboro is only about one hour and forty minutes. Since we live relatively close to the airport in Atlanta, the door-to-door travel time is close to two hours. Not a bad commute.

Thirty minutes later...

SEAL and I put on our gear to run six miles outside. Maybe it's from the flight or maybe I'm just not drinking enough, but I feel a little dehydrated before the run. This is confirmed by the fact my urine is almost brown. So, before heading out, I drink two full glasses of water. Then we're off.

About one mile into the run, I have to pee so bad it hurts. If I could cross my legs, I would. I ask SEAL if we can pull over.

"SEAL, man, I gotta pee...BAD."

"NOW? In the middle of the fucking run? On my time? Why didn't you plan your piss BEFORE the run? What the fuck do you think you're doing pissing now when this is run time? This isn't piss time."

SEAL is genuinely mad. I offended him by having to urinate on our run. So, after his thirty-second rant on the subject, I decide that I no longer have to piss anymore. I hold it in. For the next five miles of the run, all I'm thinking about is *not* peeing.

When we complete the run, I ask SEAL politely if I can urinate. "It's your time now. Do whatever the fuck you want."

One hour later...

We're at the breakfast table, one big happy family. Sara feeds Lazer applesauce, I'm reading the sports section of the *New York Post* devouring some more bananas, and a morning TV show is on in the background. SEAL slides a box of fancy granola off to the side. SEAL isn't big on rations from Whole Foods. He shakes his head when Sara offers him a bowlful. I noticed yesterday I haven't seen SEAL eating at all. I mean...as in *nothing* since he's been here. That's seven days and three meals a day and I haven't seen him eat a single bite.

But it's Sara who asks, "SEAL, are you on a diet?"

"Nah, I just like to go to sleep hungry...so I wake up hungry. Life is all about staying out of your comfort zone."

"And what's the reasoning behind that?"

My wife is very inquisitive, but not in a pushy way. She loves to learn and hear every detail when she's curious about something, and I can say with confidence that she likes to talk. Her favorite thing is having a long meal and talking about the meaning of life. SEAL is polite, but you couldn't build a dinner party around him. He looks like he's going to pull a muscle trying to converse. After about twenty questions from Sara ranging from his upbringing to what should she make for dinner tonight, I decide to cut SEAL a break and change the topic by making a suggestion.

"So what do you guys think about heading up to Connecticut to the lake house for the Christmas holiday?"

"Sounds good," SEAL says. "I want to check your security up there anyway."

"Security?" Sara says. "We don't need security; it's a private community."

"A private community? So is the White House," he answers.

The house is on Candlewood Lake in Danbury, Connecticut. Candlewood is the largest lake in Connecticut, and it's a great vacation spot. We mostly go up there as a summer retreat, but we also like to do a trip around Christmas as well. The house is in a gated community of a hundred homes.

Lawns are perfectly manicured, houses are superbly well kept, and if there is one piece of litter on the streets, it would be considered dirty. Needless to say, crime is not an issue.

"Who checked it last?" SEAL asks.

My wife looks at me and shrugs.

"That's it," SEAL says, tossing his cloth napkin on the table. "I'm going to take a look."

SEAL has a mission. He finds a clipboard I didn't even know we owned and grabs a pen.

I have a few meetings in the office, so I can't go along. I call Smith, my driver, and ask if he minds taking SEAL up to Connecticut for the night. We're scheduled to have a plumber come to the lake house the next day, so it's perfect.

"What time?" Smith asks.

SEAL is standing there with the clipboard looking at me.

"I think he's ready to go now," I say.

"Tell him I'll be there in three minutes," Smith says.

I met Smith through Jam Master Jay of Run-DMC. I knew Jay from the mid-1990s. After I wrote "Go New York Go" for the Knicks, I cofounded a company called Alphabet City. Alphabet City was a vehicle for me to sell more theme songs to teams. I was at a trade show and I saw Jay across the way from our booth. I decided to go over and introduce myself. Jay was my Ringo Starr: not the front guy of the band, but the guy that held it together. He was the guy I looked up to in the music business. We hit it off from minute one.

A month after meeting, Jay called me up. He had been working out of an office at Def Jam Records and wanted to relocate. We had created one big "war room" at Alphabet

City, and I told him he could have the desk next to mine. At that time he had just started JMJ Records and was producing a number of artists including Onyx of "Slam" fame.

Jam Master Jay had one secretary/manager and two interns who also worked out of our office. One of the interns was a young rapper from Queens named Kaeson, and the other was a rapper/boxer from Queens named Curtis. I *loved* Kaeson's music and signed him to my own private label. I didn't see the same star power in Curtis, but he helped me with a bunch of sports songs. Well, shortly after interning for us, Curtis Jackson, calling himself 50 Cent, went on his own and signed with Eminem. 50 Cent became one of the top-selling artists of the decade. BIG miss on my part.

Smith was Jay's friend, and that's how I got to know him—Smith was always at Jay's office and ultimately ended up working for Jay. Smith isn't a tough-looking guy, but you can tell he's tough. He's someone you'd let win an argument because you're afraid he'd fight you. But his exterior belies his interior. He's a gentle soul at heart.

One of the first things you learn about Smith is that he's one of those guys who always just missed. If Smith bought a Mega Millions lottery ticket today, his numbers would come in tomorrow. He's always one inch away from greatness. Smith was like the fourth member of Run-DMC no one knew about. In the early 1980s the group wanted him to be the original DJ, but he was dating a girl in Texas and didn't want to commit to the group. So instead of the meteoric fame his friends enjoyed, he ended up doing sound checks and what-ever else the group needed. Plus, he broke up with the girl.

To find out how long Smith has been just missing, you

have to go all the way back to his days in junior high. His full name is Darnell Smith, which apparently didn't single him out because there was another Darnell Smith in his class. On the playground one day in eighth grade, the two Darnell Smiths decided to play rock, paper, scissors to see who would be called "Darnell" and who would be called "Smith." And Smith just barely missed with a throw of rock only trumped by paper. He's been known as Smith ever since.

Through Jay, Smith became a close friend. After a while, our friendship felt like any of the friendships I had with the guys I grew up with except that Smith was much tougher than the guys I grew up with. After Jay was murdered by an unknown assailant at his music studio in Queens in 2002, Smith needed a job. I ran into him a couple of months after the funeral and asked him if he had a driver's license. He held up a MetroCard.

"Does this count?" he said. He was only kidding. He had a license, so I asked him if he wanted to drive for me.

"What would it entail?" he asked.

"Mostly it entails driving for me."

He's been working for me for ten years now, but he's much more than an employee—he's part of my family. He's someone I can trust and count on.

Smith drives SEAL up to the house in Connecticut. They're both going to spend the night and meet with the plumber the next morning. The plumber is going to give me an estimate on replacing some damaged tile in the steam room. I call them before I go to bed just to make sure everything is okay.

"All cool," says Smith.

But apparently it doesn't stay all cool. In the middle of the night Smith decides he's hungry and tiptoes downstairs to the kitchen because he doesn't want to wake SEAL, who's in one of the bedrooms. Smith doesn't even want to turn on the lights, so he makes his way from the bottom of the staircase to the kitchen using his cell phone for light until he manages to find the handle of the refrigerator, which he pulls open to give more light. He walks over to the counter and grabs a bag of cookies. What Smith didn't know was that we have a motion detector we turn on when we're not using the house. It goes on automatically at night. Maybe this scored some points with SEAL when he inspected the house's security. So when Smith pops the first cookie into his mouth, the alarm is triggered and sends off this earsplitting sound.

Now, Smith knows there's no intruder in the house because he triggered the alarm, but Smith also knows that SEAL doesn't know what Smith knows. Smith might have a bit of intruder experience in his repertoire, but he has absolutely none when it comes to dealing with a pissed-off Navy SEAL who might think he's an intruder.

Smith drops to the ground and crawls over underneath the kitchen table and begins to scream, "SEEEEEEEEEEE EEEEEEEEEEEEEEEEEEEEEEEAL, IT'S MEEEEEEEE, IT'S SMIIIIIIIIIIIIIIIIIITH, IT'S ME, SMITH!"

When the alarm company notified me, I called SEAL. He told me he found Smith trembling underneath the kitchen table, kneeling in a pool of spilled milk, cookie crumbs all over his face.

The next day SEAL drives back to New York and sits me down in our conference room with a report of his inspection.

He looks even more serious than when he is about to tell me what workout or run we are going to do. He's prepared.

"Man, this is fucked up. You guys are FUCKED up there."

I'm trying not to laugh. "We're on a beautiful, tranquil lake. Even the deer feel safe up there."

"The northeast windows are warped. The perimeter is exposed . . . too many entry points . . . too much glass."

I try to take a look at his report.

"This is a fucking disaster zone," he says.

"For real?"

"Man, I couldn't live in this place. NO FUCKING WAY. I can't even comprehend how you and Sara live there."

This may be the most animated I've ever seen SEAL.

"Wow . . . Well, what do you suggest we do?"

"We need to swap out all the doors IMMEDIATELY. Lock down all the nonprimary windows. AND bulletproof the glass."

"Bulletproof the glass?"

"Yep, bulletproof the glass."

"Is that really necessary? It's a lake house . . . in the middle of nowhere."

"CRITICAL . . . I'm going to contact my boy and price that sucker out."

That evening, SEAL is waiting inside the doorway when I get home. He's holding a file in his right hand. His muscles are tense. His expression is so stern it's like his face is cut from rock. He doesn't say hello. He gets right into it.

"We have two options as I see it," he says in a deadly whisper.

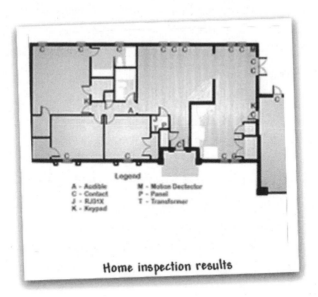

Home inspection results

"Okay."

"We can replace all the lower and midlevel windows for $450,000, or...we can say *Fuck it* and do the whole house for $785,000, which personally I think is a no-brainer."

"Seven hundred eighty-five thousand dollars?"

"Yep, but man, look. Rambo can be standing outside with an M16...and you can stick your middle finger up at him and say, *'FUCK YOU, RAMBO'*...And he won't be able to get in. This is military-grade shit. *It works.* Unless Rambo brings a bazooka, you can sleep knowing your shit is on lockdown."

Sara comes home, and I sit her down to discuss our options.

"Sweetie, SEAL gave me a quote on the security system for the lake house."

"Great, honey," she says as Lazer runs into her arms.

"He suggests we replace all our windows with bulletproof glass."

"Okay, love." She smiles while combing her fingers through our son's hair.

"It's $785,000."

My wife says nothing.

"Thoughts?" I ask with a manufactured smile.

"Well, let me ask you this, sweetie. When is the last time you saw someone walking around Candlewood Lake with an M16?"

She has a point.

"Love, can you just ask SEAL to put fire extinguishers in all the rooms and teach me how to set the alarm?" Sara smiles.

Workout totals: 6 miles

Google Me, Motherfucker

I don't like motherfuckin' freeloaders. You
better work hard for your shit or we aren't gonna
get along very well.
—SEAL

Next day...

I get a call from the plumber who went in to check the steam room tiles at the Connecticut house. The conversation went something like this:

"Hello, Mr. Itzler?"

"Yes."

"Please tell that man I did not Google you and that I would have quoted the same price if you lived in the South Bronx."

"Excuse me?"

"I don't want any trouble. But I do want you to know I've contacted my lawyer."

"What?"

"I'll take thirty percent off."

"I don't know what you're talking about."

"Okay, forty percent, damn it! Do you mind if I make a living? I have a family too!"

"Uhhh?" was all I could manage before he hung up.

It turns out SEAL had taken exception to the price the plumber quoted for the work and accused the man of going on the Internet, determining our net worth and the location of our primary residence at 15 CPW, and then trying to gouge us based on that information. The way SEAL expressed his displeasure at the plumber was to pound his fist on the tile until it began to crack while yelling: "You Googled them! You Googled them! Well, Google me, motherfucker!"

"I don't want any trouble," the plumber said on the phone. "Please. I beg you."

DAY 9

Oxygen Deprivation

Train for the unexpected.
—SEAL

New York City
23°
0600

It's only been a little over a week...nine days to be exact...
but it feels like SEAL has been living with me for fifteen
years. It's not like we're exchanging friendship bracelets,
though I do feel I understand him a bit better. He's still
spending a lot of time in his room at night, but he feels a
little more integrated into our daily lives.

Today I wake up *sore*. Or maybe stiff is the more accurate
description. I've never been one for stretching out. And I can
honestly say I've never formally stretched in all my years of
running. Not pre-run. Not post-run. It's not that I'm against
it; it's just not my thing. But today I'm going to need to figure
something out. I'm in this stiff-like locked mode and my body

can't function normally. I reach for the beeping alarm clock, and my arm can't move from a ninety-degree angle. It's stuck in an imaginary sling.

To get up, I have to clasp my hands under my legs and hurl them both out of bed. I basically have to generate enough momentum to swing my legs over the side of the bed and onto the floor. They are that stiff.

H E L P !

As I get to an upright position, I bend down and try to touch my hands to the floor. I barely get past my knees. It makes me realize that SEAL does not do any stretching either. When we do our workouts, we just start. There is no "pregame" before the runs and there are no cooldowns after. Eventually I make it out of my bedroom and see SEAL in the living room writing something down in his tiny workout log.

"SEAL, are we going to do any stretching during this whole ordeal?" I ask.

First his eyebrows arch. Then instantly his expression turns to a scowl. SEAL takes two steps closer to me and gets in real close. I can feel and hear his nostrils breathing. I think I insulted his expertise.

"What do you want, a fucking leotard? Man, we start, and then, motherfucker, we finish. That's what we do up here," he says.

Okay then.

So at 0600 today we head out to Central Park for *another* run.

No stretching.

No preparation.

My warm-up is putting on my warm clothing.

I get it.

It takes me a solid three miles to get going, but surprisingly, once we find our pace and break a sweat, my legs really loosen up. In fact, I go from feeling like a stick figure to someone performing in Cirque du Soleil—okay, maybe that's a bit of an exaggeration, but I feel good—real good. Odd. I mention it to SEAL as we run and he just replies, "Jesse, I really don't give a fuck."

As we come close to the end of the run, SEAL finds a tree with a long branch hanging straight out. We stop. SEAL jumps up and knocks out twenty-five pull-ups. No kipping. No using his legs for momentum. Just twenty-five perfect all-American pull-ups. He instructs me to do ten.

"Even if you have to stop. Do all ten."

I'm soaking wet in sweat after our six-mile run. I do six nonstop pull-ups and then drop to the ground. Back up for the last four. We return home.

I make a hot bath in my bathroom. As the warm water fills the tub I dump an entire box of Epsom salts into the water and mix it around with my hand. I have no idea if this product works, but it has been said to help muscle pain. The box says to add two scoops for every so and so gallon of water, but I'm so stiff again now that there will be no measuring. I pour the entire box in. I strip down and climb in slowly to get used to the heat. I grab a magazine, kick my feet up on top of the tub, and relax!

It feels good to be working out so hard, but I'm also starting to feel and see hints of my body breaking down. It's much harder to get out of bed in the morning, although I do appreciate my bed more, especially when I see that wooden chair. But I know I can do this.

Four hours later...

I have a meeting in my conference room. We have an idea for a new business we are calling "Sheets," and we are going through some early-stage strategy. "Sheets" are small dissolvable strips that you place on your tongue (think Listerine strip) that are loaded with caffeine, B-12, and other vitamins and nutrients. The hope is that this product could one day compete with or even replace 5-hour Energy or other on-the-go energy products. The product has unique benefits in its fast delivery system of caffeine and its portable packaging.

SEAL is in the meeting. Well...SEAL is sitting in the meeting, but I wouldn't say he is active. He is listening, but I can tell something is bothering him. He is looking at me like he is pissed off. When the group decides to take a ten-minute break to "check emails," SEAL asks if he can chat with me for a second.

Thirty seconds later we are alone in my office.

"This morning was incomplete. I got shortchanged," he says.

"Excuse me?"

"We ran. We did push-ups. We did pull-ups. But we didn't get our sit-ups in. It was an incomplete session."

"But I did everything you asked me to do," I say.

"Well, now I'm telling you that our shit was incomplete and it's fucking me up. So we are going to do them NOW."

"Now? I'm in the middle of a big meeting."

"No you're not. You're in the middle of a break."

SEAL tells me to sit my ass on the floor and then he steps on my feet.

"Lie all the way down," he says.

Then he tells me to sit up and touch his knees. I do that a hundred times. After about thirty-five I have to lie flat on the floor after every five sit-ups to get my energy and strength to do the next five. When we are done I am sweating profusely. At that exact moment, Kish comes into my office and tells me we are resuming the meeting.

SEAL and I head back to the conference room. Everyone is staring at me as sweat pours off my forehead like a faucet that has been left on. SEAL looks at the group and can clearly sense the tension.

"Jesse had some unfinished work," SEAL says. "He is ready now."

The meeting resumes.

1800 (6:00 p.m.)

Dinner.

2000 (8:00 p.m.)

Shower.

2200 (10:00 p.m.)

I hear a noise coming from SEAL's room like he's landing a helicopter in there. I knock gently on the door. Nothing. I knock a little louder. Nothing.

I'm POUNDING on the door.

"WHAT?" SEAL yells.

He opens the door and there's a camp tent on the floor. Not folded or packed away, but set up like he's going to build a campfire and roast marshmallows in the middle of my Manhattan apartment. The tent is hooked up to some type of generator with a hose. The generator is pumping full tilt. It's loud.

"Whatcha doing?" I ask casually.

"Huh?"

"WHAT ARE YOU DOING?"

"Getting ready for bed," he says.

"Ah, okay. What's that?"

"What?"

I point at the tent.

"That's a tent."

"OHHHH! It's a tent," I say.

"Yep!"

"I know it's a fucking tent, but why?"

"'Cause I'm gonna sleep in it tonight."

"You're gonna sleep in a tent? In a bedroom? On Central Park West?"

"Yes."

"Can I ask why?"

"Oxygen deprivation."

"Huh?"

"This tent deprives you of oxygen."

SEAL zips himself in and says, "I'm training too, dude. Kill the lights."

I later learn it's called an altitude-simulation tent, and

when the generator is hooked up it sucks the O2 out of the tent and helps the body produce more red blood cells. It makes your cardio system work like you're sleeping on top of Mount Everest.

I'd have to bet I'm the only guy on the Upper West Side of NYC with an inflatable raft, an oxygen deprivation tank, a tent, and a SEAL in his apartment. I get into my bed and open the window in our room. I suck in the cold NY air coming into my apartment off Central Park. It feels great. As I fall asleep I think about the lack of oxygen in SEAL's tent and again think to myself...I'm such a pussy.

Workout totals: 6 miles, 10 pull-ups, 100 sit-ups

DAY 10

The Honor Code

If you want to be pushed to your limits, you have
to train to your limits.
—SEAL

New York City
21°
0500

Sara is sound asleep. My son Lazer is asleep. Most of the
continental United States is asleep.

SEAL is *not* asleep.

SEAL is in the den.

SEAL is dressed.

Same T-shirt.

Same shorts.

He looks like he's been up for hours. Fresh. Unfazed.
Wide awake and giddy.

Me? I look like I just got off the red-eye. Tired. Worn
and pissed that I'm up.

SEAL looks like he has nothing else to do but this. Me? I have a ton of shit on my mind with Zico and making sure Coke is happy with our work to date. I'm concerned about the new Sheets product. I'm preoccupied. He is not occupied.

"You ready?" SEAL says.

"Go fuck yourself," I reply.

It's 5:00 a.m. It's way too early. I hate this.

There's generally a moment in every endeavor I undertake, be it business, love, or fitness, when I say to myself: *What the hell was I thinking?*

I'm just now experiencing that moment. Sleeping in a chair, bleeding nuts, and almost getting sued by a plumber was not what I was expecting. Sure, I pictured grueling workouts, sweat pouring off my face, and challenging my limits when I hired SEAL, but all this?

I know my friends think I'm insane right now, and they've seen me do some crazy stuff before. But this has to be at the top of the list. My whole path has been nontraditional. Any time when you live a little outside of the norm people look at you: (a) with some admiration and (b) like you're crazy. I never cared about that and I still don't. I have a complete stranger living in my apartment; I'm getting up super early and running every day when it's freezing. I think some people wished they could do it but they never would. The will to keep doing this and the will to put myself through this is what people think is crazy, and I'm paying for this, literally and metaphorically. Maybe I *am* crazy.

I know it's normal to have second thoughts about some of my decisions, but what about third, fourth, and fifth thoughts? It's pitch dark and twenty-one degrees out, for

God's sake! Maybe I'll just wrap it up, I think. Pay him for
the month, and wish him happy trails.

Then I remember the one condition I agreed to when
I hired him: Do anything he asks. SEAL built his career
around honor. At a minimum I have to honor my commitment to him.

I go change into my workout clothes.

0515

This is our push-up routine: Do one push-up then stand up
and wait fifteen seconds, then go down and do two push-
ups and wait fifteen seconds and so on, until we get up to
ten push-ups, and then we start taking thirty-second breaks.
For push-ups sixteen, seventeen, and eighteen, SEAL allows
us to take forty-five seconds between sets. What a guy! I do
sets of push-ups one to eighteen for a total of 171. Followed
by thirty pull-ups. (No time limit. As long as it takes to
knock out thirty even if I drop from the bar.) Then we go
and run quarter-mile intervals. We run the quarter miles at a
fast pace. Then we walk one minute. We repeat this for two
miles. Quarter-mile sprint...one-minute walk.

SEAL says he wants to get me up to a hundred miles of
running a week.

What? Even when I trained for marathons, my highest
weekly mileage per week was forty miles. One hundred miles
of running a week sounds like that can be dangerous. That
feels like shin-splint territory.

Meanwhile, I'm so sore from all of the push-ups I can't even wash my hair.

SEAL doesn't care, nor is he very concerned.

"If you want to be pushed to your limits, you have to train to your limits. If you get hurt, you will recover. What the fuck is the problem?"

Three hours later...

SEAL calls me into his room for a sidebar. He tells me he has to "go away" for three days. I guess he really is the "surprise-or." He's doing a seventy-five-mile race and traveling for business. I don't ask any questions.

Sometimes at night he makes calls, but I have no idea to whom or for what. I occasionally hear him talking on the phone in his room behind a closed door in a low whisper. It's not like I'm spying on him or anything, but I have to walk by his room to get to Lazer's room. I've never overheard anything he said on the phone. But it does make me wonder.

"Keep up the program while I'm gone," he says. "Do six-mile runs in the mornings and three at night. And don't forget to hit the push-ups. Make sure you get two hundred in every day. I'm going off the grid. Do this shit on the honor code."

Roger that.

I can't help but speculate where SEAL is going. Yes, he runs races. Yes, he does Ironmans. So he might be doing something like that.

But he also could be going on a secret mission. Who knows? My mind is racing with ideas.

> **Workout totals: 2-mile interval run, 171 push-ups, 30 pull-ups**

Date Night?

I'm not into sit-down dinners and fancy shit like
that. I'm into fueling up and being on my way.
—SEAL

With SEAL gone for three days, Sara plans a lovely dinner
for just the two of us. I mean, I have some input too, but
Sara wants to cook—and she's terrific. It's to be a time for
us to catch up on any topic we see fit, nothing is off limits,
and share some "quality alone time," as my wife calls it. I'm
all in. I'd taken for granted the sacrifice Sara had made. She
agreed to let someone who was basically a stranger live with
us. And although she grew fond of SEAL, we had zero alone
time.

At 3:00 p.m. she calls me at work to tell me she's leaving
for Whole Foods with a list of items for our date. She's making homemade veggie burgers, pasta, a salad, steamed spinach, and baked potatoes. My favorites!

"Six thirty sharp!!!! Be home at six thirty *sharp!*" she
says. Sara has a tendency to repeat words in sentences if they
are *really* important.

So, I leave my office at 6:00 p.m. My apartment is only a
twenty-minute walk from my office. I make it with six minutes to spare.

I peek into the kitchen: Flour. Boiling water. Veggies.
Game on!

"This looks great, honey. Can I help?"

"Please set the table and get water for us both," she says with a smile. "Dinner will be ready in four minutes." Sara pauses for a moment. "Four minutes."

In the dining room, I grab forks, spoons, knives, and two plates. I place the silverware on the side of the plates in no special order. I can't find napkins and I don't want to bother Sara. There's a powder room right off of the dining room. I unroll about three feet of toilet paper, tear it in two, and fold each section. Now we have napkins! I pull out another three feet in case we need extra. I put two of the "napkins" under the silverware and the rest in the middle of the table.

"Table is set," I yell.

"Great," she responds. "COME AND GET IT!!!!"

I walk into the kitchen with both of our plates. "This looks fantastic," I say, admiring the wonderful meal my wife has cooked. I kiss her on the forehead.

"Please, honey, you first," I say, handing her a plate.

Sara carefully constructs her meal with salad, a veggie burger, and some steamed spinach. Her plate looks like it's from a photo spread in *Bon Appétit* magazine.

"Honey, I'll meet you in the dining room," she says as she heads out of the kitchen. "I'm so excited," she adds.

As she leaves, I start filling up my plate...nibbling away during the process. One scoop of veggies on the plate...one scoop directly into my mouth.

I'm eager to sit down and eat, but food for me is fuel. I inhale...I don't eat. I think sitting through a long dinner is an inefficient use of time. I like to stand when I eat. Why not...take in the calories fast...and be on our way? With that mentality baked in my DNA, I start ingesting the food on my plate as I walk into the dining room. First a fingerful. Then a handful. Then a full-on attack. I'm starving from all the working out.

I get to the dining room table.

"Sweetie, where's your food?" Sara asks.

I look down at my empty plate.

"Did you eat all your food already????"

I shake my head no. I can't say no, because my mouth is filled with veggie burger.

Now I don't know what to do. I'm done. To me, we had a great date, no? So I sit and watch my wife eat. There's not a lot of no-limits discussion at the table. In fact, it's pretty quiet. The thought that I might have put a slight damper on our date creeps into my consciousness.

After Sara finishes eating, she wipes her mouth with the toilet-paper napkins.

"Sweetie," she says, holding the flatware between her thumb and index finger. "This is a *fork*! A F-O-R-K. Fork! A fork is an eating utensil. It's used to get food off of your plate and bring it into your mouth without getting it all over you. A fork is what *adults* use to eat."

She places the fork on the table and then holds her hand up and wiggles her fingers. "And these are called *fingers*. Fingers are used to hold the fork. They are *not* used to scoop up pasta...squeeze it into a ball...and eat it like an apple. Repeat after me: *fingers*."

"Fingers," I say.

"Are *not*," she says.

"Are *not*," I repeat.

"Used."

"Used."

"To pick up food."

"To pick up food."

Great date!

Three Years Earlier: First Date

I imagine I'm a hard guy to have a relationship with.
—SEAL

The first time I met Sara, I overheard her saying she was hosting a charity event to raise money for college scholarships for underprivileged women in Africa.

When I got back to New York, I looked the charity up. It was called the Sara Blakely Foundation, and the event was called the Give a Damn Party. The money raised was to help women in Africa attend university. I bought a table of ten on the condition it was right next to the host's table. Then I called Sara and commented on how amazing it was we were both so passionate about sending underprivileged African women to school. What a coincidence!

The night of the event, my table was indeed right next to Sara's, but I couldn't convince anyone other than one of my high school friends to fly down to Atlanta with me—there were going to be only two of us at a table for ten. So, the day of the event, I called Sara's office and they filled the table with people I didn't know. I didn't care, I was there for one reason (with all due respect to the underprivileged African women). As it turned out, I didn't get a whole lot of Sara's time that night. As the host, she didn't have a lot of time to give. But she knew I came, of course, and that was the whole point.

I must admit, while Sara intrigued me before the party, I was more interested by the time the night ended. She was even more beautiful than the first time I saw her, and she performed her duties as host with an elegant self-assuredness that was incredibly attractive. She had organized quite a night: Sir Richard Branson was there, Jewel and Collective Soul performed, but to be honest, I paid very little attention to what was going on around me. I couldn't take my eyes off Sara.

Not too long after the charity dinner, I found out, and I really don't remember how I did, that Sara had broken up with her boyfriend. I immediately emailed and invited her to go with me to the Final Four basketball championship, which was being held in Atlanta that year. She didn't know anything about basketball, but you really don't have to know anything about basketball to have fun at the NCAA Men's Finals, and she did.

Two weeks later she came up to New York for business, and I asked her out on our first official date. I told her I made reservations at a day spa and a sushi place for dinner.

"Terrific," she said.

Now, describing where we were going as a day spa was stretching it a bit. "Illegal Russian bath" was perhaps a more apt representation. I love hot saunas, and this place had a sauna so hot they made us wear felt hats so we didn't burn the roots of our hair. Sara showed up having just had her hair done that afternoon and thinking she was going to get a pedicure and a foot massage. Instead, she was led into a changing room where a Russian woman with calves the size of fire hydrants gave her a paper bottom to wear. Just the bottom.

Sara came out with her arms wrapped around her boobs to cover them up. Remember, this is our first real date.

The sauna was set for 185 degrees. Ivan the Russian therapist then comes in and performs a platza treatment on us where he beats us both with wet oak leaves to generate more body heat and takes our body temperatures to unbearable highs. Then, when he feels we can't take any more heat, he takes us to a room where he pours glacially cold water all over us. Then back to 185 degrees.

It was so romantic...

Then we went to dinner.

As I look across the dinner table in a fancy New York sushi restaurant, Sara's hair is still soaking wet and she has some mascara running down her face. The poor woman looks like she'd been boiled. However, she never once complains and we have a great time.

Sara and Jesse...Game on!

DAYS 11-12

(not counting the days I was on my own)

Enjoy the Pain

I earned it. Now I'm going to enjoy it.
—SEAL

New York City
38°
0800

I was on my own for the past two days while SEAL disappeared, and I honestly stuck with the program—Honor Code. I did six-mile runs in the morning and three-mile runs at night. And two hundred push-ups in the middle like an Oreo cookie. It was actually a bit lonely doing the workouts on my own. Not that I miss the guy, but maybe a little?

Today is no different. I did a six-mile run this morning. At 11:00 a.m. my cell phone rings and it's SEAL. He tells me he's on his way back to NYC and that he just completed the seventy-five-mile race.

"How was it?"

"Hard," he says.

"Really? Seventy-five miles was hard?"

"It had a climb," he says. "The terrain was tough."

I know SEAL well enough by now to know that if he says a race was "hard," had a "climb," and the terrain was "tough"...then it was TOUGH!

"And...I broke all the metatarsals in both feet."

Huh? Check that. Tough times twenty.

"But I finished strong," he says.

He *finished*?!

"What are you going to do?" I ask.

"What do you mean?"

"You going to go get them looked at?"

"Get what looked at?"

"Your feet."

"Why would I get them looked at?"

"'Cause they're broken!"

"Come on, man. The doctor will only tell me they're busted up. But I already know they're busted up. Why would I waste my fucking time driving to the doctor and then pay a man to tell me my feet are fucked up when I already know that? I gotta go. Call you back."

He has a point, I guess.

One hour later...

I'm in my home office when I get an email SEAL sends while he's in the car on the way to the airport:

From: SEAL
To: Jesse Itzler
Subject: On my way

Training will go on.

The guy breaks every bone in both his feet but can still run? Training will go on?

11:00 p.m.

The front door of the apartment swings open. It's SEAL. He has a key, but since he's been living with us, we hardly ever lock the door during the day. What's the purpose? Today is no different, and he opens the door.

As he makes his way in, SEAL is walking like he's stepping on broken glass. He's limping and in obvious pain. He's not wearing any shoes, and his toes are really messed up. SEAL is missing the toenail on his right big toe, and he has a few blisters that look like his toes swallowed giant red grapes. OUCH.

"Man...that looks bad. You gotta do something for it," I say.

"Nah, I'm just gonna sit on the couch and enjoy the pain," he says. "I earned it. Now I'm going to enjoy it." He starts to laugh to himself.

At first I thought that maybe he wanted to impress me and create this crazy persona. Like overplay some of this stuff for effect. But now as I look at his battered feet, I realize that there is no overplaying this kind of thing. There is no effect. He really means it. He really wants to enjoy the pain.

Next day

I'm at my office getting caught up on work when I get a call from Mark Rampolla, the CEO of Zico. He gets right into it.

"A lot of people in the Zico office are reading your blog about SEAL," he says.

"Awesome," I say. "Thanks for sharing."

"Yeah, they can't believe you are doing this. You're nuts. You must be getting in great shape, and you must be exhausted."

"Yes...and definitely YES!"

"Well, anyway, we want to know if SEAL would endorse Zico. You know, use it at races and talk about the product, et cetera?" he asks as his words hang in the air like a puff of white smoke.

I feel like telling Rampolla that SEAL doesn't really talk, but I say "great idea" and I will ask. "Call ya back," I say.

I hang up and tell SEAL about the conversation.

"You are blogging about this?"

"Yeah, at first I just sent it to a few friends who love to work out, but now it is catching on. And it's kind of spread a little bit, but just a little bit," I say.

"Okay, cool, but I don't want any part of that shit. None."

"Any interest in endorsing Zico?"

"I race for me. I don't race for products, Jesse. I race for me."

We leave it at that.

Dinner

1730

I hear the *Rocky* theme playing in SEAL's bedroom. It plays once and then I hear it again. Then again. And again. Then the song repeats approximately thirty times. What the fuck is he doing in there?

I choose not to knock on the door but can tell there's something serious going on in that room. I can almost feel heat coming out of the door. I'm curious.

Finally, after the thirty-first time of the song repeating, SEAL walks out. He is soaking wet and leaving puddles of sweat all over the floor.

"You okay?" I ask.

"Twenty-five hundred push-ups, motherfucker. Yes, I am okay."

Sara walks into the room as she too is curious. However, I can tell her curiosity suddenly changes to concern. Something is bothering her. Really bothering her. I can see it on her face she's trying to tell me what's on her mind...without talking. She's sending me some kind of husband-wife telepathy through her eyebrows and expression, but I'm not getting the message clearly. I wonder if I get points for at least knowing she's trying to send me subliminal Morse code?

Then her eyes slowly shift from my eyes to the floor. They go there in slow motion, taking my eyes with them. It is there that I see a puddle of sweat growing larger by the second on our silk Oriental rug. It's the same rug that has been passed down from generation to generation and was given to Sara by her grandmother. With every passing second the puddle spreads out like it's raining all in one spot... dead smack in the middle of the family rug. As SEAL sits on our couch, sweat pours off his nose and lands on the rug in a steady flow.

I immediately go to the bathroom and get two towels, one for SEAL and one to place on the rug. I'm in trouble.

Sara calls me into our bedroom.

"Don't ever let that happen again," Sara says to me. "I'm dead serious." She says it in a tone that is way scarier than anything SEAL has said or done to me to date. It even rivals my mother's silent treatment. "Never," she repeats.

Thirty minutes later...

It's 8:30 p.m. and we are on our first workout of the day (well, at least I am). We do a series of push-up sets one to eighteen, for a total of 171. Then we head downstairs to the gym. Residents have 24/7 access. It's pitch dark when we get down there but I immediately flip on the gym lights.

I never ran on a treadmill until I met SEAL. I'm an old-fashioned, lace-on-the-kicks-and-run-out-the-front-door kind of runner. SEAL thinks a treadmill is a good training tool because it's controlled. Yeah. Like Chinese water torture.

He has me walk for five minutes at a 12.5 incline at a

fifteen-minute pace. Then, he reduces me to a 3.0 incline, but makes me do:

1/4 mile: 9:30 pace
1/4 mile: 6:50 pace
1/4 mile: 9:20 pace
1/4 mile: 6:40 pace
1/4 mile: 9:20 pace
1/4 mile: 6:30 pace
1/4 mile: 9:00 pace
1/4 mile: 6:20 pace

Approximately three hours later (11:30 p.m.)

SEAL tells me it's time for some sit-ups. It's like we are cramming for a test trying to get our daily double workout in before midnight.

He always makes sure I have proper form. As in all the way up and all the way down, as fast as you can do them, or they don't count:

44 unassisted ("Unassisted" means no help with lots of yelling.)
1 minute rest
44 unassisted
1 minute rest
44 unassisted
1 minute rest
Total: 132

Push-ups:

15X @ 7 sets (on the minute): 105 total
Rest 1:30
12X @ 9 sets (on 50-second mark): 108 total
Rest 1:30
10x @ 10 sets (on the 45-second mark): 100 total
Total: 313

I'm wiped out. But I'm so wired from endorphins I can't fall asleep. Never in my life have I worked out late at night. I'm used to knocking it out first thing in the morning.

SEAL comes in and tells me to set my alarm for 0730. We are starting at 0800 sharp tomorrow, so I set my alarm for 0745. I want those extra fifteen minutes of sleep. It dawns on me that SEAL doesn't have an alarm clock. Yet he never oversleeps; he's always up when I get up. In fact, now that I think about it, I've never actually seen him asleep. I've never seen him yawn, never even seen him stretch or even seen him close his eyes for any length of time. This dude is a robot.

> **Workout totals: 5-minute walk on a steep incline, 8 miles (2 miles of which were intervals), 132 sit-ups, 484 push-ups**

DAY 13

Sick Fuck Friday

Every day is a challenge, otherwise it's not a
regular day.
—SEAL

New York City
21°
0800

It's been less than eight hours since I did my 484 push-ups. Five hours since I fell asleep. When I get up, SEAL is already up. I mean, *wide awake* up. He tells me he has been outside surveying our running route, checking the terrain, feeling it out.

"The terrain?"

"It's not a regular day in Central Park," he says.

"No?"

"Nope. Nobody's smiling. There are only a few stragglers out running. One guy is walking a dog. Saw one delivery guy."

"Okay."

"Nah, man, it's not okay," he says. "Only the loonies are out there today, bro. Only the demented...It's sick fuck Friday."

I'm not sure what he means.

I walk out the front door as SEAL limps.

We set out to run five miles at an eight-minute pace, but SEAL wants the run to be mostly hills. He settles on running the small back part of Central Park by 110th Street. So we run uptown and when we get there, we do the small loop of the 110th Street hill. The hill is only about a quarter of a mile up, but it's steep. To hold an eight-minute pace is *very* challenging.

As we ascend, my shoulders kill from the 484 push-ups yesterday. I mean *they are killing me.*

My arms dangle from my sides as I run to ease the sharp pain in my shoulders. They're not sore. I'm beyond being sore. I'm trying any technique to ease the pain. *Nothing works.* At the end of our run, I bend over huffing and puffing. My arms hang like they're dead. I need to give them a day off.

"How are your shoulders feeling, bitch?" he asks.

I don't even respond.

"Tonight more push-ups. I'm gonna test your shoulders," SEAL says, limping past me. "Be ready."

1:00 p.m.

I decided to work from home today, so SEAL is in his room "chilling out" and I'm in my room making calls. I can't lift anything (even my cell phone) because my shoulders

hurt so much, and I'm not exaggerating. SEAL walks into my
room.

"I'm going down to the gym to get a quick workout in."

"Okay," I respond.

Two hours later

SEAL returns to the apartment holding his hands up to show
me his palms. They look like he fell off his bike and braced
his fall with his hands. They're battered.

"What happened?"

"I knocked out my pull-ups."

"How many you get?"

"I did five pull-ups on the minute for two hours."

"You just did six hundred pull-ups? Just now? Just like
that?"

"Roger that. So go fuck your bullshit shoulders," he says.
"Whatever you got going on, someone else has more pain.
You gotta learn how to fight through it. No matter what it
is . . . Think about someone else and take a suck-shit pill."

I think he means a suck-it-up pill, but I don't question
him. "Suck-shit pill" sounds good to me!

2200

SEAL has been in his room the entire afternoon and evening.
I have no idea what he's doing but he has not once come out
and looked for me. Is he mad? I didn't dare to bother him;

who wants to wake up a sleeping giant? As the night creeps in, I realize I'm exhausted. Plus, I need to let my shoulders recover. I crawl into bed with my clothes on and fall sound asleep at 10:00 p.m. I'm zonked out.

At 12:30 a.m. my alarm goes off. Now, I know I didn't set my alarm. I know my wife didn't set the alarm. And I'm damn sure Lazer didn't set the alarm.

"Trick or treat," SEAL says.

He's sitting in my room on a chair four feet from my bed in his running gear. I think he's eating a banana. I rub my eyes to make sure I'm not dreaming, and, sadly, I'm not. I'm more freaked out than the first time I saw *Silence of the Lambs*. The only way this could be worse is if he told me to put the lotion in the basket.

He walks over to my side of the bed, bends down so his mouth is basically inside my right ear, and starts quietly whispering the lyrics to the Geto Boys hit song, "At night I can't sleep, I toss and I turn..."

I pretend like I'm sleeping, but he repeats that line over and over...louder and LOUDER...until I finally get up.

We head outside. It's the middle of the night. Well, actually, it's the start of the middle of the night. Actually, it's one hour past midnight.

It's about twenty degrees but feels like minus-five degrees with the wind. We do a three-mile run around the lower loop of Central Park, forty jumping jacks, then ten push-ups, and repeat. We do twenty sets of the jacks and push-ups in fifteen minutes. That's eight hundred jumping jacks and two hundred push-ups in *fifteen minutes*!

There was not a living thing stirring in Central Park while

we trained. Not a civilian. Not a police officer. Not even a squirrel. I'm bruised and battered. The only way I could feel worse is if SEAL made me carry him home.

I don't give him any ideas. I just want to be warm. Who trains at 1:00 a.m. outside in the middle of winter?

When we get inside, I take off all my clothing and throw on some dry boxer shorts and an old short-sleeve tee. Then I grab my winter jacket from the foyer closet and put it on. I was so damn cold from the run my jacket is the only thing that is appealing to me. I zipper it up to my chin and climb into bed. I know I'm at 15 Central Park West, but it feels like I'm on a mission in Serbia in the winter. I look at Sara; she's in the fetal position in the middle of the bed spooning with her pillow. I throw the hood of the jacket over my head and pull it up until it covers my eyes. Lights out.

> **Workout totals: 8 miles, 800 jumping jacks, 200 push-ups**

Lady in the Honda

Everyone is a potential threat.
—SEAL

SEAL and I head up to my lake house in Connecticut. I need to make sure the pipes didn't freeze and take care of some odds and ends. After we check everything off the list, we get ready to head back to New York. I ask SEAL if he'd mind doing the driving so I can get some work done.

"Roger that."

"How are your driving skills?"

"I'm well trained."

We start driving back to the city. SEAL apparently is a defensive driver. I note that he even uses the turn signal to pull out of the driveway. I nod left to confirm which way to the interstate. I grab my phone to check emails and then give him a nod when we need to take a right at the fork. I snatch a pen from the glove compartment to take a few notes. Eventually we get on the main road.

SEAL points his index finger at the first car we pass. Then he does it again to the next car. Like his hand is off the wheel pointing. Again he does it. Plus, he's talking to himself in a low melodic voice mumbling.

"Mblamblamblam," he mumbles and points.

"The pointing thing, is that some kind of—?"

"Yeah, it's a driving technique. You need to point at the target. Every target," SEAL says, pointing at an eighteen-wheeler.

"But these are just commuters. Guys coming home from work."

"That's what they are to you. To me, they're targets."

I check out the next car we pass. It's a mom with two kids in the back watching videos. SEAL points at her.

"You have no idea what the lady in that Honda can do," he says. "You have no clue what her reaction time is. You have no inkling to what that lady is thinking. Honestly, you don't know shit."

We sit in silence for a minute.

"Man, you wanna drive?" SEAL asks, sensing my discomfort.

"No, not at all. I've just never seen a technique like that. Where you point at every approaching car."

"You're too trusting, man. It just takes ONE pissed off mom. BAM. It happens that fast. A fucking nanosecond. Reach for your phone and KA-POW, you're blasted. You need to think prevention and stop singing that Elton John SHIT, Jesse!"

"Elton John?"

I have no idea what he's talking about.

"All cylinders, baby," he says. "This is no joke. This shit is like a video game behind this wheel. You can get gobbled up real quick. You need to have your shit tight on the roads out here."

DAY 14

Fireman's Carry

If you can't do the basics, you can't do shit.
—SEAL

New York City
22°
0945

SEAL has about ten pills in his hand, and he throws them all back in his mouth in one giant handful. He then takes a swig of water and opens his mouth.

"AHH," he says, and they are gone.

I'm not sure what SEAL is taking. Vitamins? Medicine? Anti-radiation tablets in the event of an attack? Who knows? All I know is he is taking horse-size pills in large quantities at odd hours.

"Let's stay inside for forty-five minutes," SEAL says.

"Why?"

"You'll see." SEAL chuckles.

We take the elevator down to the basement where there's

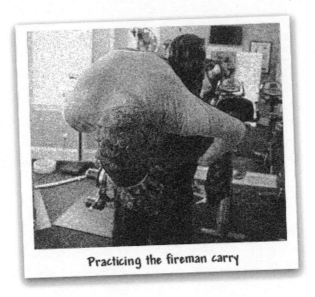

Practicing the fireman carry

a hallway that's about thirty yards long. SEAL says we're going to do fireman carries.

"It's a basic military workout," he says.

I have to throw SEAL over my shoulder and run thirty yards in the hallway of the basement, drop SEAL, do thirty-five reps (four count) of flutter kicks, flip to my knees and do twenty push-ups, then we switch and he carries me. We are to repeat this fourteen times.

By the twelfth repetition, I'm messed up. Like really screwed. This is up there with the worst I've ever felt in my life.

Carrying SEAL was brutal, but being carried by him was way worse. Imagine all the blood rushing to your head from being carried upside down. Plus, SEAL's shoulder is digging into my torso.

During one of the reps, the elevator opens and a resident

steps out of the elevator and into our hallway. I recognize her, but I don't know her name. I've seen her on TV and I think she's a real estate mogul or something, but at this hour, who cares? I realize the people in my building must think I'm crazy. They must be wondering what's going on. This is a building with fancy handbags with poodles living in those bags. We do not fit in. They must want to know why Rambo is living in their building.

Anyway, she can sense the insanity, and she looks at both of us, scared and yet curious. She walks unusually fast toward the gym. It's almost like when you see someone on the street and they suddenly realize they aren't where they want to be and quickly change pace.

"This looks a bit intense," she says as she walks by me and into the gym.

A little intense? I'm thinking. How about crazy intense?

3:00 p.m.

I walk into my office and SEAL is sitting by my desk on the phone. He rocks back and forth in my comfy swivel chair.

"It's Garnett," SEAL says to me.

"Yeah, man, be cool," he says as he hangs up the phone.

Apparently SEAL and Garnett have stayed in touch. I have no clue how either of them got each other's contact info, nor do I know what those guys are possibly talking about, but it makes me smile that they are connected.

SEAL gets up and I sit at my desk and power up my computer.

"No need for that now," he says.

"What do you mean?"

"We are going to check in on your burpee progress. Same drill."

"Come on, man, I got shit to do today."

"So do I. Take your shit off and get started."

I strip down to my boxers.

One...two...three...ninety-nine...one hundred!

Ten minutes and twenty-seven seconds! I feel myself smile.

2218

I get home late from a New York Knicks game. I walked the twenty blocks to the Garden directly from work. Today I had multiple meetings, multiple conference calls, and had to put out multiple fires at work, plus the fireman workout killed me this morning. Then the burpees. And then the walk to the Garden.

I'm somewhere between the front door and comatose when I hear "Let's run eight."

"C'mon, man...It's over. Let's just do early tomorrow."

"Okay, if that's what you want," SEAL says, looking at me like I'm a pussy.

When SEAL wanted to become a SEAL, he weighed 290 pounds. You can't be 290 pounds and be a SEAL, he was told. So he lost 105 pounds in less than two months. I know it sounds impossible, but he lived on fresh fruit and water and worked out like a madman (naturally!).

In SEAL training, you're subjected to something called

"Hell Week." Over a five-and-a-half-day period he was allowed only two hours of sleep. His class had just finished exercises in freezing water when their instructor ordered them back in. A SEAL in training standing next to him stared vacantly. There was no expression in his classmate's eyes. They were hollow. SEAL called it "the Look." The classmate turned and walked away. He quit.

SEAL looks at me like I have the Look.

I man up. We get our shit on. It's twenty-two degrees outside. I'm mad as hell that I'm doing this. When we walk out of the front door, I turn to SEAL and say, "FUCK YOU."

"Let's go," he says.

11:00 p.m.

We start running to the Hudson River.

Before he pushes the button on his watch to start the run, I plead to do only four miles. He says eight. Miraculously we settle on six. We start.

I can honestly say there's *not one single person* other than us running at 11:25 p.m. on the West Side Highway. *Not one.*

As we run I notice my shoulders are in extreme pain from this morning's workout. I run with my arms dangling by my sides. That lasts for a half mile because this type of running style kills your thighs. (Try running fast for a half mile with your arms like this if you don't believe me.)

Now I have a choice: severe shoulder pain or running like an asshole with my arms dangling. I opt for the running-like-an-asshole look partly because there's not a soul on the streets to see me.

During the fifty-three-minute run, SEAL and I don't say one single sentence to each other. Not a peep. It's like *Night of the Living Dead.* He only says two words the entire run:

"Turn around" at the halfway mark.

Three miles back in silence. It's midnight when we finish.

"Tomorrow starts at oh six hundred," he says as we walk into my building. "Get some sleep."

> **Workout totals: 6 miles, 100 burpees, and 14 fireman carries**

DAY 15

It's All About the Push-ups

If you're gonna do 'em, do 'em right.
—SEAL

New York City to Atlanta
28° to 49°
0600

I walk into the kitchen and SEAL has a look on his face that I have never seen. It's a cross between furious and confused. It's scary. He's having a heated debate...with himself.

"Let's add some extra mileage today," SEAL says. "Nah, let's knock out a slow eight," he says back to himself. "Nah, fuck that. Let's knock out a slow six and then do two AFAWC."

When he says it, it sounds like "AFLAC" from the commercial with the duck, but it's not. It's AFAWC: as fast as we can.

"Yeah, motherfucker, we're gonna do six miles and then do two AFAWC."

It's about twenty-eight degrees outside today. However, today I decide to dress more like SEAL does and only wear shorts and two T-shirts, but double up on the hat and gloves. Without the extra layers, I'm feeling light and we fly on the run.

The first six miles are at an 8:06 pace, then SEAL takes the pace to 7:29 for the last two miles. As soon as we hit the six-mile mark, he says to me "sub seven thirty" and speeds up. He doesn't even look at his watch; he just programs his pace like someone would program a car to a certain speed on cruise control.

When we get home, I peel two bananas and dip them in honey. I one-bite them and am done in about ten seconds. I grab a Zico and hit the shower. We just flew through that run, and I'm feeling great...not just about the run, but how much I'm improving. How I have been able to hang in there.

The funny thing is, SEAL has not complimented me once, which is fine. It's not like I need his validation, but it would be encouraging. That said, I'm genuinely proud of myself. It's like this experience is a personal test of will... it's the ultimate "can I make it?"...and so far I think I'm winning.

I note it as such.

Five hours later...

We head to LaGuardia for a Delta flight to Atlanta. Sara wants to check in at Spanx HQ tomorrow, and we decided yesterday that we would all go. Although we have access to Marquis Jet, we often fly Delta. SEAL doesn't seem to mind either way, and he is totally indifferent about where we train just as long as there are NO FUCKING SURPRISES. I give him at least a twenty-four-hour heads-up before any travel now. I'm looking forward to the flight as it represents two to three hours where I can just read and listen to music. SEAL just sits and stares on a commercial flight. I can't even guess what he's thinking about. Truthfully I don't even want to know. So I'm usually not factored into the equation. I get comfortable in my seat and wonder what I should read first.

But today's flight is different. SEAL wants to talk.

"So tell me your shit," SEAL says.

"My shit?"

"Yeah, your shit."

"Okay," I say, reclining my seat back as far as it can go. "What story do you want to hear: (a) The Big Red Chicken; (b) Don't Let Them Boo You; (c) Larry the Coconut Guy; or (d) 1-800-PLAYMATE?"

"Who the fuck wants to hear a story about a big red chicken?"

"Well, it's not really about a chicken," I say.

"Keep your fucking chicken stories to yourself," he says. "I go with D, motherfucker...D."

"Well, I moved from LA back to New York in the summer of 1992. After I realized there would be no second album," I say.

I came up with an idea to start my own record label so I could sign my own artists. I partnered up with my friend Spit and we called it Riot Records. To be honest, that sounds a lot more impressive than it was. First of all, I didn't have enough money to rent an apartment so I was sleeping on friends' couches. Second, the first deal I made didn't exactly go according to plan.

The artist we lined up was a woman named "Crystal," who was confirmed to be a centerfold in an upcoming magazine issue. Mike Ross had suggested her to me. Maybe I should have known better since he turned her down. When I first talked to Crystal on the phone, I asked her to sing "Happy Birthday" to me as a kind of audition. The sound that came out of the phone was like someone with bronchitis trying to sing "Old McDonald Had a Farm"...while being strangled. But that centerfold thing...

So...I agreed to do it! Again, get that foot in the door... figure it out later!

Crystal already had some good marketing ideas in place. She'd worked out a deal with the magazine to publicize a contest where if you bought the record, you were given the chance to win a date with her. This promotion was going as an insert in the magazine that would be distributed to hundreds of thousands of people. I thought the idea guaranteed strong sales just to pimply-faced teenage boys alone.

One weekend we took Crystal out to the Hamptons summer share house where we were staying. She definitely didn't get the memo because she walked around the whole time topless. I'm not even sure she packed a top. Now, she's like a fifteen out of a possible ten. None of my college friends had ever been exposed to anything like her. She was like the hot chick they invented in the movie *Weird Science*. All of the pent-up sexual energy in the house made me think this was going to be a great idea.

My friend Spit's parents had a place in the mountains, and I moved all of my recording equipment into their house. The idea was we would block off a solid week and record her album with her at the house. One night after recording, we joined Spit's parents for dinner at their dining room table.

Everything went along just fine: the usual small talk and niceties. Then Spit's father brings up the Miss America Pageant that was on TV the night before.

"They asked some tough questions of the finalists," he said. "One was who they thought the most influential woman in the last century was."

"That's easy," Spit's mom said. "Eleanor Roosevelt."

Crystal didn't say a word. She was the perfect guest, albeit one with thirty-eight-inch perfectly shaped breasts that stretched the limits of the white Nirvana T-shirt she wore, but was quiet at dinner. Then, right on the heels of the name Eleanor Roosevelt coming out of Spit's mom's mouth, she decides to weigh in.

"ELEANOR ROOSEVELT???? I would *not* say she was that influential," she said.

"Why's that?" Spit's mom asks.

"Well, all she did was fuck a president," Crystal responded.

I thought Spit was going to choke on the Eli's baguette he was chomping on. Mrs. Spit looked like someone had just taken a crap on the dinner table in front of her; but Mr. Spit,

God bless him, sort of cocked his head and let his glance drop ever so slightly down on Kurt Cobain's face.

"She's got a point," he said.

We eventually made Crystal's record. While she waited for the magazine to come out, she decided to make some extra money dancing at a famous Manhattan strip club. One night she bumps (literally) into Baba Booey from *The Howard Stern Show*, who falls headfirst for her. Between dances, he tells her he wants her to come on Howard's show. She gives him my number. When he calls me, he tells me there is one condition: She has to come on the show completely naked. "From the second she gets off the elevator, she has to be nude." After consulting with Crystal, we booked the appearance.

I figured I'd milk this appearance for everything I could, so I got a 1-800 number that had the ability to take three hundred orders a minute. We'd charge $9.99 for the CD, which we'd split. Crystal would promote the record on the Stern show, give out the 800 number, and I was going to sit back and watch the orders roll in. Boo-ya!!!

The day Crystal went on the show I was home listening on the radio. Spit took Crystal to the studio. When Howard saw her walk in naked he went crazy—he said he'd never seen anyone so hot…EVER! It couldn't have gone any better—Howard's fully engaged, really funny, the interview even goes past the allotted time. By the time they played her song, I'd already started counting the money in my head. Then Howard asks her to tell his listeners how they can order the record.

We must have rehearsed what she was going to say the

night before twenty thousand times. Twenty thousand times. I did everything but tattoo the 800 number on her...well, her palm. But from the radio all I heard was the disturbing sound of nothing.

Howard Stern: "Is there a number they can call, Crystal? Crystal? Crystal?"

Silence.

I was screaming the number at the radio. Finally, Crystal begins to speak. But my relief quickly turns into utter disbelief. To a national audience on the highest-rated show on radio, she gives out *not* the 800 number that we practiced but my personal *home* phone number to call and order her record, which started to ring immediately.

Oh, my God. I thought.

Although I tried, any attempt to keep up with the demand was futile. In the few calls I did answer, the comments ranged from junior high stupid, to sexual offender stuff. I just stopped answering.

My phone rang without pause for three solid hours. Then, just when it seemed to slow down, the show aired on the West Coast. The onslaught happened all over again. We didn't sell a single CD, I had to change my phone number, and we ended up not releasing her album.

SEAL has a hint of a smile on his face. I think he likes the story.

"All the profit I made from my own album, which was about $50,000, I'd lost in a matter of months with Riot Records," I say.

"Poof," SEAL says. "Are you still friends with Crystal?"

1800

We land and head to baggage claim in Atlanta. A friend of mine, Lisa, comes over and says hello. She didn't realize we were on the same flight; neither did I. I do a quick introduction to her with SEAL.

"I know who you are," she says.

"That so," SEAL says.

"I read Jesse's blog," Lisa says, and she gives us a coy smile. SEAL still isn't smiling. He just looks at me and gives me a silent grunt and then looks back at Lisa.

She extends her hand and he shakes it.

"I know who you are too. You were sitting in seat fourteen C," SEAL says. "The guy next to you was dark-skinned and reading *Reader's Digest*. I'm aware."

Lisa looks at me with a "holy shit . . . what the fuck" face.

2200

After we get settled into the house in Atlanta, SEAL summons me to the living room.

SEAL believes push-ups are the single best exercise for strength. He also believes proper form is the key. You get more out of ten push-ups the right way than thirty done improperly.

Proper form: back straight, ass up slightly, neck straight (don't drop your neck). Go down and break ninety degrees with elbows, and make sure your chest hits the floor. Go all the way up (until arm is fully extended).

We begin doing our one to eighteen push-ups and then eighteen to one. So our first set has one push-up with a fifteen-second rest; then we do two push-ups with a fifteen-second rest. All the way to eighteen and then back down to one. In case you're counting, that's 342 total. So SEAL has me do eight more for good luck. That's 350 push-ups.

We finish around midnight.

> **Workout totals: 8 miles (2 AFAWC) and 350 push-ups**

Perfect Position

I'm on alert. High alert. Even when you don't
think I'm on alert, I'm on alert. Even right now,
I'm on alert.
—SEAL

Sara and I have plans tonight for dinner. Friends of ours own
a popular restaurant in Atlanta called 10 Degrees South,
and we have a 7:00 p.m. reservation. The restaurant has a
South African safari motif and cuisine. It's refined—no paper
napkins, no bare feet—but it's not pretentious. We ask SEAL
if he wants to join us.

"Roger that."

We drive to the restaurant.

I'm in jeans and a button-down. Sara wears a dress.
SEAL is in a black T-shirt.

He takes the seat on the far side of the table so his back
is against the wall. From there he can see the entire land-
scape of the restaurant and notifies us that he has the exits
staked out.

"I'm in perfect position," he says.

Our table is fairly close to the kitchen door, which is
heavy. It makes a small boom every time it closes, which
makes SEAL clench and bounce up.

"Yo, you okay, man?" I whisper. "That jumping thing..."

"Yeah, I'm cool. Just them loud noises, man," SEAL says.

"The door?"

"Yeah, the door. It's freaking me out."

"It is?"

"It sounds like a fucking explosion or something. It's loud. It's unpredictable," he says.

"Should I have them leave the door open?"

"No. I'll block out the sound."

"You can do that?"

"Of course. You could explode the fucking Goodyear Blimp in here and if you're zoned in, you can block that shit out."

Sara and I look at each other but don't say anything.

A waiter comes over and hands us menus. He points to the specials on the board and takes our drink order. I've never seen SEAL drink anything other than water in a restaurant. At home he likes to drink special, "military-grade" shakes "that you can't get online." It's a combination of protein and carbs and comes in chocolate and vanilla. That's his "meal." You order it through a special website.

SEAL glares at the waiter as he takes our order.

"SEAL, what's up?"

He whispers, "Man, this motherfucker right here. I don't trust that dude."

"Our waiter?"

"Yeah, whatever he says he is," he says.

"I'm pretty sure he's just our waiter."

"Nah. I've seen this movie before, man. I don't trust that motherfucker at all."

"What makes you feel like that?"

"Well, for one, his whole pretty-boy act: his smile, his gear, his walk, his silly-ass laugh, the grin, that bullshit attire."

"I think that is his waiter's outfit."

"Fuck that," SEAL whispers. "Guy's a threat."

"Wow. I don't see that at all."

"Really?" SEAL's eyes go wide. "You don't? Man, he knows what time the cash comes in and out. He knows when this place opens and when it closes down. He has ties to all the delivery guys. You trust the fucking delivery guys here, Jesse?"

"I haven't given it a lot of thought."

"Oh, you haven't, huh?" SEAL is now livid. "You see who brings the shit into this place? The delivery guys. They know all the patterns. MAN! Just keep your eyes on that dude. That's all I'm saying, Jesse. Keep your eyes on that dude."

I look over at our waiter. Come to think of it, he does look a little sneaky.

"Everyone in this place is capable of something. Remember that, Jesse...EVERYONE."

Our waiter returns with our food. I keep one eye on him as he sets down the butterflied prawns. Sara is now looking at our waiter like she doesn't trust him now either.

DAY 16

Stay Lite

You can get through any workout because
everything ends.
—SEAL

Atlanta
55°
0700

As Sara heads out to the Spanx headquarters, SEAL and I
head out for a run in Atlanta. The route is simple: three miles
down Peachtree Road, turn around, and come home. It's a
beautiful day in Atlanta, fifty-five degrees and sunny, and it's
warming up fast as the sun starts to climb. SEAL takes his
shirt off and we take off.

Peachtree is a main road in Atlanta. There are like ten
different Peachtrees and I'm not sure which one is which, but
this is the main one. I'm still not familiar with the streets here,
so no matter where I have to go, I just take this version of
Peachtree. I know eventually it will get me where I need to go.

It's almost rush hour here and the street is starting to get crowded. Cars are backed up at red lights and traffic is slow moving. The sidewalk we're running on is roughly two feet from the oncoming traffic. If I look into the window of the cars we pass on the run, I can see the blemishes on the faces of the drivers. We are that close.

I can feel the eyes of the drivers in traffic looking at us. It's making me uncomfortable and also making me run faster. SEAL, well, he couldn't give two shits. He is so locked in on the run I don't think he notices one single car. But he has to. He has to know that he stands out like a sore thumb, right? He is a V-shaped mountain of African-American muscle running up Peachtree. Everyone is looking at him.

When Sara gets to Spanx, she hears rumblings throughout the office about the specimen running down Peachtree. Sara's office has about two hundred women, half of whom just passed SEAL on their morning commute to work. So you can imagine how quickly word spread throughout the office.

Buckhead, where Spanx is headquartered, has a pretty typical cast of characters. Men wear suits, basically all have the same haircut, and drive the same three cars—Mercedes, Range Rover, or BMW. So seeing SEAL wearing only short flimsy running shorts looking like every inch of his body was meticulously carved out of stone...seemed a little out of place to say the least...and caused quite a stir.

My phone rings...It's Sara. She says in a whisper, "Honey, everyone here is talking about SEAL, wondering who he is and where he came from. What do I do? Do I mention the 'specimen' is living with us?"

1430

After a late-morning flight, we arrive back in NYC and head home.

SEAL greets the FedEx guy at the door. It appears Christmas has come early for him, or maybe for me. He ordered me my very own fifty-pound metal-plated weight vest for push-ups and to "increase the level of difficulty" of my runs. You've got to love SEAL. I didn't even know my runs needed a higher degree of difficulty.

"It's on, motherfuckers!" he yells, jumping up and down as he opens the package. "It's on!"

I don't think I've seen SEAL this excited—ever. He takes the vest from the box and puts it on. It fits perfectly. The thing looks like a suicide bomber's vest. If he walked into a bank wearing it, people would dive under their desks and give him the combination to the vault without him even asking for it.

"Today we test it out." SEAL grins.

We have one vest and have to share it, so I go first.

We do a three-mile run with the extra fifty pounds strapped onto my body. The vest is uneven, so the weight shifts from one shoulder to the other. It's brutal and makes it hard as hell to run.

It's so painful the three miles take thirty-three minutes. Each step is torture.

SEAL asks for the vest. We switch off and I'm free. He's so happy you'd think he's putting on the Masters' green jacket.

We run three more miles. It takes him/us 22:30.

Total run: 55:30.

I come home and fall asleep on the couch. I literally can't move.

Sixty minutes later...

"Grab the vest," SEAL says.

"You're joking," I say.

"Actually, I'm not," he says. "Grab the vest, fucker."

I clutch the vest.

"I can't," I say. "I need to watch Lazer." Sara has a work function tonight, so my parenting duties are doubled.

"Bring him," SEAL says. "All three of us are training today."

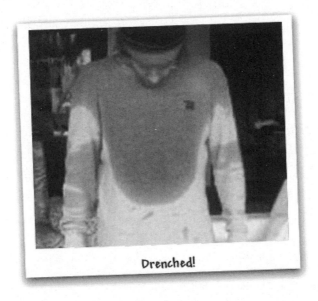

Drenched!

"But he's eighteen months old," I say. "And it's only twenty degrees outside."

"Bring him," SEAL says firmly.

I bundle up Lazer and we start running.

I'm wearing the vest. It weighs as much as a safe. SEAL pushes my son in the stroller next to us.

I go two and a half miles wearing the vest. It takes thirty-one minutes.

I've been on a thousand runs in my day. I've run eighteen New York City marathons in a row. I've done ultra-marathons of a hundred miles. This is one of the most brutal runs of my life. No question.

I pull over every hundred yards and drop to my knees and adjust the vest. I try to shift the weight to save my shoulders. The heft kills me. I shift again. It doesn't help. People in the park are starting to stare. They want to know what the fuck is wrong with me. They also want to know what the fuck two grown men in weight vests are doing pushing a baby stroller in twenty degrees.

I wish I knew ... I wish I knew ...

At this point I'm out of options; the shifting provides no temporary relief anymore. I'm done.

"What the hell are we doing? This is ridiculous. Can't you see this is killing me?"

"Relax, Jesse, you need to know that everything ends. Just do this shit and it will end."

We switch. SEAL puts on the vest.

We run another two and a half miles.

FAST.

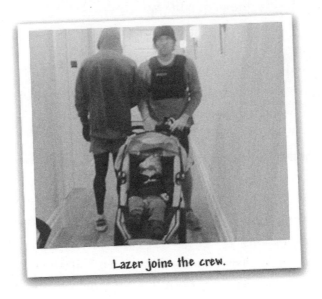

Lazer joins the crew.

8:00 p.m.

I'm starving. I feel like I need at least ten thousand calories. Maybe that is because I burned ten thousand calories today.

"SEAL, I'm ordering in some food. What'dya want?"

"I'm good."

"Come on, you gotta be starving."

"Nah, man, I'm good. I'm staying light."

I order in dinner for three and start to eat and I'm still hungry as I'm shoveling food in as fast as I can. SEAL grabs a banana and some almonds on his way to his room.

"See ya in the a.m.," he says.

With a mouthful of food I try to enunciate "See ya," and food flies out of my mouth as I do.

A few minutes later, Sara calls to check in. She asks to talk to Lazer who babbles "mama" into the phone. I pull the phone away and am so grateful Lazer hasn't learned the words "help me!"

"All is good here, honey...we've got it under control."

> **Workout totals: 17 miles (5.5 miles in 50-pound vest)**

DAY 17

Suicide Bombers

If a motherfucker looks crazy, usually the
motherfucker is crazy.
—SEAL

New York City
18°
0500

Sting is not in the gym when we walk in, but Bob Costas is.
He's on the treadmill watching the news on the tiny screen.
I see Costas a lot in the gym and love chatting sports in
between sets.

SEAL starts setting up the gym like a wedding planner
would set up a reception. He lays out the bench press bench
in one section, then grabs the curling bar and moves it to
another section. After a quick assessment, he spreads out a
rubber mat for sit-ups in another location. Before you know
it, we have a variety of circuits perfectly laid out.

He tells me the routine and we start:

Dumbbell bench press: 15 reps at 35 pounds, 12 reps at 40 pounds, 10 reps at 45 pounds, 8 reps at 50 pounds, and then 6 reps at 55 pounds.

Then, we do seated rows: 15–12–10–8–6 (medium weight). 51 reps.

Then, we do military press: 4 sets of 10 (medium weight). 40 reps.

Then, we do triceps pull-down: 15–12–10 (light weigh). 37 reps.

Curls: 15–12–10 (25 pound dumbbells). 37 reps.

Sit-ups: 50…one minute rest…then 50 flutter kicks: 50 four-count flutter kicks (basically do a flutter kick for 4 seconds…that equals 1).

Costas is now ignoring the television and is focused on us. I fly through the workouts with *zero* talking. The workouts are starting to have a definite precision to them; meaning… SEAL is really focused on my form, and I'm finally getting comfortable with my technique. I think Costas has noticed the improvement. At least he has in my head. I grab my towel and we leave the gym.

SEAL pats me on the back and says, "Nice work."

My first real compliment!

0650

I have to be at work at 7:00 a.m. for a breakfast meeting (well,
the guy I'm meeting will have breakfast, I will be having
fruit), and SEAL makes me wear the weight vest to the office
today. He wears the one he borrowed from the guy at the
gym. Mine's under my jacket. SEAL just wears his vest over
a T-shirt. We walk around Columbus Circle over toward my
office on Park Avenue. It's not a bad walk, but today we stand
out. I think we look like suicide bombers from a J.J. Abrams
movie. Shoulder to shoulder, black guy, white guy, down Park
Avenue looking like we're going to blow some shit up just for
the sake of blowing some shit up. We are walking with some
purpose down the street.

"We'll do this from now on," SEAL says.

I'm a bit freaked out. Not because of the weight of the
vest, but because I'm thinking we are going to get stopped
by the police. September 11 is still on people's minds, and
we don't look at all sane. I'm worried that we will get asked
to freeze and instructed to put our hands up and someone I
know will see me. We keep walking.

We walk to work every day we're in New York, and something curious happens during these walks. Most of the time
I spend with SEAL is either working out, getting ready to
workout, recovering from working out, or talking about working out. Little of it is enjoyable. It isn't all misery (although
much of it is), but there isn't a whole lot of human interaction.

However, during the walks to work that changes a little.
Just a little.

Today he asks me what I do with my money. Meaning, do I invest it? In real estate? Stocks? He had saved some money from being in the military and is curious as to what to do with it. I thought that was very "human" of him!

Rather than go into detail about my portfolio, I give him a quote that my wife says about money. "Money is fun to make, fun to spend, and fun to give away. That sums it all up." He *loves* it! He looks at me like Sara had written the Gettysburg Address and I was reciting it. "Fuck yeah, Sara," he says.

So, I give him more. "Sara also likes to think of money as a big magnifying glass. If you are a good person before you had money...then money makes you an even better person. If you were a charitable person before you had money... then money makes you even *more* charitable. But if you were an asshole before you had money...well then, money makes you an even *bigger* asshole."

"That's some fucking real poetic shit right there," SEAL says. "Sara doesn't play."

We keep pace.

As the small talk disseminates, it becomes obvious to me that SEAL is very suspicious of some of the pedestrians on the street. Out of nowhere he says, "Cross the street" and then "I don't like the way things are looking on Fifty-first today."

I'm like, *really*?

One day on the walk to work, SEAL made us go all the way over to the West Side Highway, down to 57th Street, and then back up around to my office. This added an extra twenty minutes to the walk.

"Let's stay away from Trump Tower today," he said. "Trump been in the news too much lately."

We also talked some sports on our walks, and he put up
with the ten thousand questions I asked him every day. I'd
ask him ten thousand and he'd ask me none. He couldn't
relate to my business accomplishments, and there's nothing
I could do physically that would impress him because he's
already done it longer, faster, and harder. So there was really
nothing he could ask me.

When SEAL asks about money, it seems a little strange.
I can tell it's purely out of curiosity. It's not like he's angling
for anything. He just doesn't understand how I live the way
I live. Can you imagine what it would be like if we switched
places for a week? Like one of those Disney movies where we
somehow magically switched bodies. I don't think either of
us could function right away, but I'm sure by the end of the
second act we would both learn valuable lessons from each
other.

SEAL would laugh at how simple his life was and how
complicated mine was. I would have a call list for the day, a
schedule, my bag, appointments, calendars, and such, and he
would literally grab his military card and $50, and that was
all he needed for the day. That was his whole existence. He
didn't have a car, a house, or anything to tie him down. If I
fly someplace for a weekend, I always have to check my bag.
He showed up at my house with a backpack. For thirty-plus
days. One backpack. We have closets full of shit we never
use, millions of pictures we took that we never look at, stacks
of files that collect dust. He's a master at keeping it simple,
and I have to say his simplicity looks attractive to me. I sort
of want what he has, but I still want what I have.

SEAL has me thinking a lot about my own life as well as his. Mine seems ultra-calculating these days. It gets really complicated. You get pulled in a lot of directions. I know it sounds cliché, but the journey really is more important than the destination. Once you get where you're going, most of the magic drains out. I could really see myself as a minimalist, just taking life wherever it leads me.

I like my walks with SEAL in the morning.

2:00 p.m.

I throw two MorningStar veggie burgers in the microwave and cut up some raw carrots as a side for lunch. SEAL is in his room on the phone. I'm not sure who he is talking to, but he is being intentionally quiet. Before he can hang up, I have already inhaled both the veggie burgers. I throw two more into the microwave.

"You're done," SEAL says. "Time."

We head down to the gym and start our second workout of the day with an interval run on the treadmill. I grab a towel and leave it on the handrail of the treadmill because I know I'm going to need it:

Walk 5:00 at 12 incline (3.5 speed)
2:30 at 6.2 speed
2:30 at 8.7 speed
2:30 at 6.3 speed
2:30 at 8.8 speed

I grab the towel and wipe off my forehead. I'm starting to drip. My sweat is landing on the treadmill and making each stride super-slippery. I'm convinced I'm going to fly off like George Jetson did when I start sprinting.

2:30 at 6.4 speed
2:30 at 8.9 speed
2:30 at 6.5 speed
2:30 at 9.0 speed
5:00 walk/cooldown
1–30 push-ups (Time: 41 minutes)

Halfway through the run I start to feel like my Morning-Stars may come up. I'm cramping a bit but figure I can run through it. As the cramp moves from the side of my stomach to the center, I think it may be gas. I push. It is gas. I push a bit harder and a loud "fahhhhh" blasts out of my ass. It's like a thundercloud has burst out of me.

SEAL looks and me and says, "Fahhhhh," in the same exact pitch as my fart. I keep running but start laughing hysterically on the treadmill. SEAL is standing there just staring at my pace on the electronic dashboard of the machine. No smile. No laugh.

Ninety minutes later... around 3:00 p.m.

I want to pick up some gifts at Barneys, a fancy department store on Madison Avenue, for Sara and Lazer as the holidays are coming up soon. SEAL comes with me because SEAL comes everywhere with me. SEAL suggests we run there, but I tell him I don't want to be sweating while we're shopping.

"Well, we can run home then," he says.

"But we'll have all of the shopping bags and stuff," I say.

"Fuck it. Let's run there," he says.

So we run crosstown to Barneys. Since I know we are going to be holiday shopping on the Upper East Side of New York, I want to look somewhat respectable. So, I'm running in the nicest running outfit I have. I'm holding my credit card in my hand and a $20 bill in case we need to cab it back. By the time we get into the store, I've got a nice sweat going. SEAL looks like he took a cab there. He is unblemished.

I say to SEAL, "Let's make this fast, let's just go to the jewelry section." My wife certainly doesn't need anything, but she definitely needs to see the effort. If there is one thing I've learned about marriage, it's not the gift that counts, it's the effort. That's kind of like SEAL, I guess.

As we look at the jewelry in the glass case, I ask SEAL what he likes. "Man, this shit doesn't make any sense to me. Who would want a gold snake on their wrist for a few weeks' salary?" He has another point.

"I mean you work one hundred twenty hours and you go buy a bracelet? Shit is crazy to me."

And another point.

I pick up a few items (effort!), and ask the salesclerk to wrap them and throw the gifts in a bag. I have the $20 in my hand, but obviously we run home. Straight crosstown with a Barneys bag hanging from one arm. Bonus miles. Again, crazy. Two grown men running through Manhattan holding a Barneys bag.

> **Workout totals: 3 miles (25 minutes of intervals on treadmill), 465 push-ups, 50 sit-ups, 50 flutter kicks, and SEAL circuit: dumbbell bench presses, seated rows, military press, tri pull-downs, curls**

DAY 18

The Difference Five Minutes Can Make

Don't get too comfortable. Ever.
—SEAL

New York City
21°
0700

Miracle of miracles. We take the morning off.

"Hey, Lazer," I say to him in his highchair. "What do you think if Daddy stays home from work this morning to play?"

Lazer's smile lights up the room. First we start with his action figures and then we get into some serious block building. I haven't thought about anything other than how to build a higher tower in hours.

"Should we knock it down?" I ask Lazer.

And before the grin on his face is fully formed, the tower of blocks comes crashing down.

"Let's build it again," I say.

1145

SEAL walks in. He reminds me that it's almost noon and I have a 12:30 p.m. meeting today with the Zico sales team. I kiss my son on the forehead with a big smooch and head out the door with SEAL.

I've got on a winter coat and my Knicks knit hat. SEAL has a T-shirt and jeans on. His shoulders are angled up into his neck as we walk to work and his hands are in his pockets. He must be cold. This is unusual for him, I've never seen his body look like this before.

We are on a direct walking path to my office today, which is also unusual. Sara convinced SEAL the weighted vests were a bad idea so we look like civilians today. I guess SEAL doesn't think there are any imminent issues en route. Or maybe he feels the urge to change our pattern so we are less likely to be detected. Whatever the case, it's a normal person's commute—a direct shot.

As we hit the corner of 57th and Broadway, we wait for the WALK sign. "You ever worry about all these meetings you take? Like what if the direction isn't going the way you want it to go?"

"Never let them boo you," I say.

One of SEAL's eyebrows arches.

"No matter what, you can never let them 'boo' you. You have to control the situation."

His shoulders immediately drop down into a normal position and he asks, "What do you mean?"

"Can I tell you a story?" I ask. The WALK sign illuminates.

"Sure. Just as long as it's not about a big red chicken," he says.

"Okay, well after my video debuted on *Yo! MTV Raps*, I went on tour to support my CD. My first single, 'Shake It Like a White Girl,' was starting to get national radio play. While I was on the road, I got a call from Mike Ross. A promoter had reached out and asked if I would perform at the Increase the Peace charity benefit in Atlanta. Apparently, the promoter was getting African American artists and Caucasian artists to come together and play one big benefit show. Some of the biggest acts were confirmed. I guess Vanilla Ice was booked that day, 'cause they called me as the 'Caucasian' representative.

"The show was at the Georgia Dome in downtown Atlanta and they bused in about twenty-five thousand kids from all over Atlanta to attend. I'd known the crowd was going to be tough, but they were worse than I'd anticipated. The kids were unruly. There were fights in the stands. They were throwing shit at the stage. They had to keep putting the house lights on to control the audience. And...they booed everyone...I mean, EVERYONE. It was *insane*.

"Shortly before I was supposed to go onstage, LL Cool J was on. They had to move up his start time because he had another gig later that night and he had to fly out. The fans in Atlanta...they booed LL. I was like, 'If this crowd is booing LL, I'm in *big* trouble. Real big trouble. They are booing L and I'm supposed to go up and sing my song, "Shake It Like a

White Girl"?' I couldn't figure out how I was going to get out of this thing. I did not want to go on. I was physically sick.

"When the MC of the event introduced me, it was even worse.

"'Ladies and gentleman…all the way from Los Angeles, Californ-I-A…give it up for my MAIN MAN…JESSE JAYYYMEEES.'

"Silence.

"Radio silence.

"I could see the whites of the eyes of the fans in the first row. They were pissed. I don't know at what, but they were pissed. Before the crowd could even get the 'B' in 'Boo' out of their mouths, I came up with a crazy idea. My label had given me some free T-shirts to give away. I grabbed the cordless mic from the soundman backstage but also grabbed a pile of a hundred or so T-shirts and took them out with me onstage.

"'Atlanta, Georgia, do you want some FREE SHIIIIIT?' I yelled to the crowd.

"'YEAH!' they screamed back.

"'You all want some T-shirts up in the back section?'

"'Yeah!'

"'To my left?'

"'Yeah!'

"I kept throwing out T-shirts until they were all gone.

"Then, before anyone could even react, I said 'Good night, Atlanta. Love you guys and enjoy the show. Color Me Badd is on next.' Then I walked off the stage.

"Didn't sing a word. But I didn't get booed either. Remember when you told me to 'control my mind' the first day you moved in with me, well, I'm telling you in business... 'control the situation.'"

"Yo, Jesse man, motherfucking JESSE! You see!!! That's what I'm talking about, motherfucker. That's what I'm talking about," SEAL says, as we get to the entrance of my office building.

1300

When we get up to my office, I ask SEAL if I can have some privacy for a moment. Usually he sits on the couch and watches me type emails during the day, but this afternoon I want to be alone. I want to just sit in my chair and think.

So, SEAL pulls up a chair and places it right in front of my office and closes the door. He sits in front of it like he is guarding the royal palace in London. If anyone has to ask me a question about Zico, well, they will have to get past SEAL first.

That fact that we took the morning off makes me feel like I'm on a week's vacation. I recline on my chair and start to think about all that has happened with SEAL. I'm reliving the past days in my mind when... zzzzzzzzzzzzzzzzzzz—I'm out. Like saliva-drooling-out-of-the-side-of-my-mouth asleep. Three hours later SEAL comes in and wakes me up.

"Let's get out of here," he says.

7:00 p.m.

As SEAL and I walk into my building's gym that evening, my twenty-four-year-old nephew, Yoni, is leaving. He uses the building gym often and I run into him like this from time to time. It's always nice to see him. Typically it's a slap of the hand, a hug, and a quick catch-up. "How's Lazer?" and "How's work?"

Yoni is in amazing shape. When he moved to New York from Florida eighteen months ago, he weighed 240 pounds. I don't know if it was the New York women or what, but something clicked in his brain and he decided to get in shape. He is now about 170 pounds and *ripped*. He has run several marathons and is a workout junkie.

"Come on, Yoni, join us," SEAL says. "We're doing push-ups."

"I wish. I already ran this morning and swam just now, but thanks."

SEAL whispers something in my nephew's ear. No idea what he says, but the expression on Yoni's face goes from happy-go-lucky to furrowed and pasty. Whatever SEAL said it manipulated my nephew. He decides to join us.

"This is what we're gonna do," SEAL says. "Twelve push-ups every forty-five seconds for twenty-two minutes, then fifteen pull-ups, two minutes rest. Then twenty push-ups, three pull-ups (five sets). Then a hundred flutter kicks."

"I should have left five minutes earlier," Yoni whispers.

After working out, we all grab a quick bite at the restaurant in our building. It's a bit fancy, but we grab a table in the back and order some light appetizers. The conversation is centered on Yoni and how far he has come with his training. It escalates.

SEAL somehow convinces Yoni that he should quit his "bullshit" job running social media for a big hotel chain and join the Navy. *And*...my cockamamie nephew has bought into it. It escalates even further. Now SEAL is convincing him he can pass the Navy SEAL training and become a SEAL. He is going over the requirements and the basic fit test. It escalates even further.

"Fuck this. Let's start this shit right now."

These two knuckleheads decide to head out for a run.

I go upstairs and about ninety minutes later SEAL returns to the apartment.

"Where's Yoni?"

"Not sure. He fell back about a hundred meters at mile four."

Ninety minutes later...

Yoni walks into the apartment. He looks like a pile of split fuck. He has vomit on his fleece and he is super pale. He looks dehydrated.

"I think I'm more of a social media guy," he says.

> **Workout totals: 364 push-ups, 30 pull-ups, 100 flutter kicks**

DAY 19

My Shoulders

You can always keep going.
—SEAL

New York City
28°
0700

We head out to the loop around Central Park. I really want to stay in bed and watch the beginning of the *Today* show with Sara, but I'm in a great rhythm with SEAL and don't want to let up. Plus, there is only about a week or so left of his time with me.

Today's goal sounds simple: 6.1 miles at a sub-eight-minute pace, with no mile over eight minutes.

Before I'm halfway through the run, though, my shoulders feel like I'm giving the rapper Fat Joe a piggyback ride. The pain is ridiculous. That's what thousands of push-ups in ten days will do. I literally (no BS) can't swing my arms as I run because my shoulders hurt so badly.

So I run the last three or so miles with my arms flailing. I look like the scarecrow in *The Wizard of Oz*. The slowest mile in the first five is 7:45. The last one is 8:08. SEAL looks at me like I left him on the battlefield.

Four hours later...

I have a meeting with the brass of a major hotel chain. I'm not really sure what the meeting is about, but my friend Kirk Posmantur set it up because he thought I could help the chain. Kirk owns a company called Axcess Luxury & Lifestyle, and he is the king of connecting dots. If Kirk says it's worth a meeting and exploring, then it's worth a meeting and exploring.

I ask SEAL to join.

There's no need to change, mostly because SEAL has nothing to change into. Rather, we throw on our ridiculous-looking weight vests (SEAL is again insisting on us wearing them) and we head to the meeting from the apartment. When we arrive, we are greeted by Kirk and four other guys in suits, and they look a lot smarter than me. I am definitely not prepared for the meeting. In fact, I'm a bit nervous.

"Nice vest," Kirk says.

"Oh, this old thing." I laugh. "I just threw it on."

They are so confused.

I immediately introduce SEAL and explain that he is living with me for a month and tailing my every move.

"Wait...like a Navy SEAL seal?" the Brooks Brother guy asks.

"What kind of training?" the Prada suit dude asks.

"Like lives in your house?" the sweater vest pipes in before I can answer any of the questions. All these guys want to do is talk about our workouts and why I hired SEAL. These guys are looking at me like I just invented the Internet. They're *blown away*. It's like when a stock on the New York Stock Exchange is halted and no business can be conducted. They're obsessed with our dynamic. They keep asking questions.

Two hours pass and it's a question-and-answer frenzy. At the end of the meeting they say to me "If you have any ideas for us, let us know, we want to do something with you."

It's like SEAL is a secret weapon. He's the best closer. I'm slowly realizing how appealing SEAL is to others. Men in suits are fascinated by a guy like SEAL. His work ethic. His workouts. His history. So...indirectly they are becoming more interested in me.

1900

Tonight is my company's holiday party. And of course SEAL is invited. I'm not sure if he wants to go, but he's coming. He deserves to be here; his mere presence practically signed Kevin Garnett for us. We all have a lot to celebrate. It's been a great year.

The party is a low-key dinner and all twelve employees attend. I'm worried a bit about how SEAL will interact in the social setting. I mean, there is a good chance he will sit there and not say a word. He can be like a sphinx. When he comes to work with me every day, he never talks to anyone. EVER. Never logs on to a computer. Never reads a paper. He just sits there until it's time to go. It's like having a piece of artwork in my office. I know he's trained to go off the grid, but it was wild. Not only to me but to everyone I work with. SEAL once told me that when he came back from a mission, when everyone would sit around and smoke and decompress, he would go running. After a twenty-four-hour mission, he would work out.

As it turns out, I don't have to worry about SEAL interacting with anyone tonight because he's on a food mission. I realize SEAL's eating habits are more complicated than I originally thought. For two weeks he hardly ate at all, except for his military-grade shakes. But at dinner this evening, he eats like a wood chipper. Steak, fish, fruits, vegetables, you name it—it goes down the hatch. Everything except dessert.

"Why would I want to waste the calories?" he says.

My employees seem a little looser than they usually are during the workday. Maybe it's the cocktails. They are all obsessed with SEAL. They ask him a million questions and get one-word answers back. They're intimidated and intrigued. It's like everyone wants to sit next to him, but nobody wants to sit next to him. Most of the people at the party have been following the blog. So they know what to ask but are afraid to ask it.

"Um, excuse me, do you mind telling me what you think has been the hardest workout so far?"

"I'm sorry to bother you, but can you explain what 1-18 is?"

"If you don't mind, would you tell me the Boston story?"

My employees are asking questions like we're in the conference room with a new potential client pitching us a product. It keeps going. And he keeps eating. When all is said and done, SEAL's food intake constitutes 75 percent of the dinner bill for the night.

Amazing.

On another note, we're serving sake at the party. I like sake.

I do a shot. Then another. And another. All the way to eight (well, maybe nine!).

It's on!

First drink(s) in eighteen days.

Best I've felt in eighteen days!

SEAL is totally cool with it. He is letting me do my thing and enjoying his hall pass as well.

The euphoria doesn't last.

When we get home, I definitely need to sleep. I was up at 6:00 a.m., worked out, had an eleven-hour workday followed by the party and all that alcohol. I'm toast. I can't wait to go to bed. My body and brain are both in agreement. The day should be over, but my gut tells me it isn't. It's sort of like when you're in third grade and look out at the one inch of snow that fell overnight. You *hope* school will be canceled, but you *know* better. So regardless of what my brain and body are rooting for, I make my way to my bedroom to get my shorts and sneakers.

SEAL smiles. "You know we gotta do it, right?"

"Yes."

I'm buzzed, and doing push-ups when you are buzzed is a whole different kind of thing. I actually think it may be easier at first. The first ones are funny. It's like you don't really know you're doing them, with the alcohol and the up-and-down push-up movement mixing to form a more intense buzz. But as you move on, that buzz turns to an I'm-fucked feeling.

I fight through the fucked feeling and we do ten push-ups on the minute for twenty minutes. That's another two hundred down. It's easy to write "two hundred" on paper, but it's another thing to do them. I have no idea how many push-ups the average forty-plus man can do, but I'm guessing around twenty at one shot. Doing two hundred is a *big* number. It is not easy.

I get into my bed and throw *SportsCenter* on. I'm fucked up.

> **Workout totals: 6 miles (sub-8-minute-mile pace) and 200 push-ups**

DAY 20

Start When the Second Hand Hits

If you're hungry, run faster. You'll be home quicker.
—SEAL

New York City
32°
0600

I get out of bed and head into the kitchen. It is pitch dark outside and cloudy. It looks brutally cold, but the thermometer says thirty-two degrees. I look out of my window onto Columbus Circle and there is nobody outside. It looks like an old barren movie set. SEAL is already in the kitchen sitting on a stool at our island. Just sitting.

"We are going to focus on the basics this morning. Push-ups and sit-ups. It all starts with the basics," SEAL says.

It's true.

My time with SEAL has convinced me the days of the

fancy gym memberships are numbered. Things like CrossFit and street workouts are going to prevail in the future. All you really need to do is get your push-up and sit-up routine consistent, and you can see amazing results.

I have another philosophy. You can be fit without being healthy, but you can't be healthy without being fit. Meaning…you can be in great shape on the outside, but if you don't eat great and don't take care of your insides, you aren't necessarily healthy. History shows us there were plenty of athletes who were in great shape but suddenly died of a heart attack. Balance is key.

I also believe being in really good shape takes a combination of many components. For starters, you have to be strong, but you also have to be explosive, flexible, capable of running stop-and-go sprints and running long distances. You need the full package.

So, back to basics.

I do ten push-ups followed by as many sit-ups as I can until the second hand on the clock hits 12 again. Then I start the push-ups and sit-ups again. We repeat that for thirty minutes nonstop. By the end of the workout, my core muscles, chest, and triceps are cooked. Plus my heart rate is up in the mid-150s.

The full package.

1300

My friend Bryan Fried comes over to hang out for a few hours. I've known Fried for a long time, and he is part of my

"Wonderful Wednesday" group, six friends who run together every Wednesday (hence the name). He is also a professional cyclist and in great shape. I think SEAL is in his room, but I told him I had a friend coming over, so I assume he'll come out to say hi.

"This beats your first apartment," Bryan says, getting comfortable on my couch.

"It does," I say. "But there was some charm to that place."

"When did you live there? Ninety-three?"

"Yeah."

It was on 60th between First and York. This was long before they renovated the 59th Street Bridge area. It was actually the mecca for transvestite prostitution. Every night coming home from the bars was an adventure. The first week living there I didn't even make eye contact. It only took a week or two for all of the prostitutes to know that Spit (my roommate) and I weren't looking for dates. Well, I should say we weren't looking for those kinds of dates. In no time we coexisted, but the crib wasn't exactly the Ritz-Carlton. We had to walk up 162 steps to get to our 150-square-foot apartment. The kitchen and bathroom were one room. There was no bedroom. I slept in a loft space with a six-foot ceiling. I couldn't sit up in bed and had to walk up these little steps to get to my mattress. I'd roll just to get into bed. And looking back, I had absolutely the best time living there. It was like sleeping on a ship. I paid $350 and Spit paid $417 a month. We lived there for two years.

My office then was the apartment living room.

I'd bought a television and it came in a huge cardboard

box. So I flipped the box upside down and that was my desk. It took up half the apartment. I'd write all of the phone numbers, dates, and appointments on the box. The only rule in the apartment was you couldn't drink on my desk. That box was my whole life. I had it forever. It was so organized. I knew where everyone's phone number was. I knew every appointment.

I loved living as a struggling artist; my mind-set was a creative eat what you kill. I was enjoying the fact that I was even in this position. I worked all day hitting the phone or studio if I had a job and then at night I was hitting the bars.

Just as Bryan and I are getting situated on the couch, laughing and talking, SEAL walks in the room to shake Bryan's hand. I think SEAL wants to show off his work on me to date as he says, "Let's knock out a quick five-minute round of push-ups."

Fried and I agree.

SEAL pulls out his watch and we begin. We do ten push-ups on the thirty-second dial. By the time we are three minutes into it, Fried is down to seven. I keep pace. Five minutes pass and we're done. I'm able to do them all. Fried is cooked. SEAL is proud of his student.

2100

SEAL pulls me off the couch where I am comfortably watching ESPN.

"Let's do a cooldown" are his exact words.

To SEAL, a cooldown is an eight-mile run. To me, a cooldown is the last thing I want to do. I put on all my shit and give Sara a kiss. Although we have been doing this for weeks, she can tell I'm tired and have already had multiple workouts today. She can tell I'm pissed. "Honey, this is really ridiculous. You're overdoing it."

We run through Central Park into Harlem up around 125th Street and start to head back.

There are three specific highlights from the run:

1. Three miles into the run I ask SEAL if he has $2 (the only words we have said to each other all run). He says, "For what?" I respond, "I haven't eaten all day. I need an energy bar or a banana." He says, "We have five miles left. If you are hungry, run faster. You'll be home quicker."

2. SEAL hears a dog nearby in the woods while we are running. I didn't hear a thing, but apparently SEAL has extrasensory hearing. SEAL says under his breath to himself and to the invisible dog, "Try me, mother-fucker. I mean it, try me." Let me be perfectly honest; he said it in a way where it sounded like he *wanted* the dog to attack him. The dog was smart; we never saw him.

3. There are millions of people in New York City. Literally millions. Yet tonight we only saw one other person running in all of Central Park. We're home at 10:25 p.m. At the doorstep to our building, SEAL says to me: "It's not what you do, it's when and how you do it. It's all about the conditions. Remember that."

Ten minutes later...

We have to hustle because we need to get to the airport and go down to Atlanta for a lightning-quick trip. Sara has a meeting in the morning and has asked us to keep her company. I want to stay in NYC and work, but SEAL reminds me, "You're not in control here, bro," and he's right. If my wife wants to roll to Atlanta...we roll to Atlanta. So we fly out at midnight. The plan is to go there and fly back in just twenty-four hours.

> **Workout totals: 8 miles, 400 push-ups, and 550 sit-ups**

White Van

I can sit still for hours. Waiting.
—SEAL

The next morning I see SEAL sitting absolutely still on the windowsill of our Atlanta house. The sun is still coming up. He's staring out at something. Maybe he's watching the sunrise, but I doubt it. He's dead silent. He doesn't even acknowledge me when I enter the kitchen. His eyes are locked onto the empty street outside. Staring...

I open the refrigerator and pour some juice into a glass. I intentionally make it noisy. No acknowledgment. Zero. He doesn't flinch. Staring...

"Everything cool?"

"Not really," SEAL says. Staring...

He pauses for a moment. He might see something.

"This shit is starting to get to me. Like it's makin' me uncomfortable. Real uncomfortable."

"What?"

"You tellin' me you haven't noticed?" SEAL asks. Still staring...

"No? What?"

"That white van?" he says.

I look outside. There's nothing. The street is empty, but it looks like it's going to be a nice day.

"Man, this van keeps driving by. It's like they are toying with me, bro. Like they're clowning me," SEAL says.

I look back out the kitchen window. I still don't see anything.
"Where?"

"NO...NOT NOW. Usually around oh-two-hundred when I'm on lookout," he says.

"Lookout?"

"Yeah, lookout. Last time I was here at night I was sitting outside monitoring and the van creeped up. They were looking at the house. Fucking creepers."

SEAL continues to stare out the window. Not once does he look at me.

"I didn't get a read on the plate," he says. "But I'm onto them." SEAL ponders his thought. "By the way...you need to install an infrared camera at the west side of the driveway adjacent to the mailbox. IMMEDIATELY. It needs to be angled toward oncoming traffic. We can plant around it to make it blend with the bush. I got a guy that can install ASAP. That way we can't miss 'em. We've been breached, dude. Do not ignore this."

"Breached?"

"You've seen the van, right?"

"Actually, I haven't seen any cars in front of the house."

SEAL turns to me with a blank, cold, motionless face. He's pissed. *Really pissed.*

"It's a VAN, bro. It's not a car. It's a FUCKING VAN. The kind that looks like it's gonna do some shit it ain't supposed to be doing." SEAL stares back out the window again, at nothing. "Does the van think I'm some kinda fuckwad?"

I don't think I'm supposed to answer the question.

"I'm gonna camp out on this motherfucker," he says.

"Camp out?"

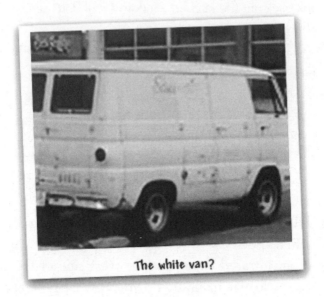

The white van?

"Fuck yeah! I'm gonna camp out and wait for his ass."
SEAL pounds his fist against the wall.

"At night?"

"Not at night. EVERY NIGHT," he says. "I'll be out there
on a lawn chair every night till that joker pulls up again.
Then I'm gonna blast a high-beam light directly into his eyes
and storm the vehicle. I'm gonna corner this fucker. I'm done
playing defense."

SEAL pauses in thought, then says: "The thing is...he
has no idea I'm even playing defense right now. He's probably thinking to himself, HO-HUM, the Itzlers are asleep.
But NO HO-HUM. The Itzlers are NOT asleep. The goblins
are awake in the Itzler house, bro." He cackles. "The goblins
are WIDE AWAKE!"

And still staring...

DAY 21

One Rep at a Time

I don't like to talk to strangers. Actually,
I don't like to talk, period.
—SEAL

New York City
19°
0900

We're back in the city, and we head out to do a modified loop
in the park. SEAL tells me we are going to run ten miles
today in reverse order, meaning four miles this morning and
six miles at night. Usually we do a longer run in the morning
and a cooldown at night. Today we do the first four miles
at an eight-minute pace. Four-mile runs are becoming easy
breezy.

I've spent countless hours with SEAL running by now,
and we haven't spoken a word pounding the pavement for
days. Complete radio silence when we run. *Nothing ever
said.*

"Hey, SEAL, what do you think about when you run?"

"Finishing."

And he does. It's like he is able to block out all the clutter in his head and the world, for that matter, and just focus on the task at hand. Say what you want, but the dude has mastered the art of being present. There is something really cool about that.

As for me, I have a million things running through my brain…Sara, Lazer, work, meetings, Zico/Coke, training, the pipes freezing, blah blah blah. It's like there's a six-lane express highway running through my brain, and traffic is coming both ways. It's very hard for me to get my thoughts, worries, and ideas out my mind. It's a bit overwhelming and stressful.

However, with SEAL around, I am learning how to be more present. It's primarily because I have to. If I don't, there is no way I will be able to finish the tasks at hand. I just go one step at a time. One rep at a time. And when I'm done, I worry about the next step or rep. I'm finding that there's some crossover to my life as well. Now I finish the first thing on my list with 100 percent focus and then attack the next.

Thanks, SEAL.

2030

After a light meal of plain pasta with nothing on it, sliced carrots, cucumbers, and a glass of water, it's time for the second half of our reverse run. I would prefer to wait about an hour for my food to digest, but SEAL doesn't want to lose an hour of his life. So, we go.

As we ride the elevator down to the lobby of my building, I explain that I feel bloated. I like to run on an empty stomach and have a very hard time running with anything in me. That goes for races of any distance including marathons. Pre-marathons all I ever eat are bananas. So I ask SEAL how he approaches nutrition during his long races.

"I need calories when I'm running that long. I have trained myself to be able to eat while I'm running. I can take in six hundred to a thousand calories an hour, no problem. But it takes getting used to."

I hear the same thing from other ultra-marathon runners. They have become capable of eating large amounts of food during their races. Dean Karnazes, a legendary runner who put ultra-marathoning on the map, is famous for eating pizza during some of his longer runs. He actually orders and has the delivery guy meet him on the course so he can get the pizza and eat it during the race.

All that is good, but none of it is working for me as we start to run. I can feel the sustenance in my stomach bouncing. I'm belching every couple of strides. It's like the pasta, carrots, and cucumbers have set up a picket line in my belly and are protesting against one more step. We're not even at mile one yet and I feel heavy and sick. SEAL couldn't give three shits and keeps pace. In fact, I think he senses my discomfort and speeds the pace up a bit to make me feel even worse.

At around four miles I somehow figure out that if I breathe exclusively through my diaphragm, it feels a little better. I incorporate an unorthodox breathing style for the last two miles and make it home.

It takes about an hour for my stomach to settle down, but the run is in the books.

Another ten-mile day. Book it!

> **Workout totals: 10 miles @ 8-minute-mile pace**

DAYS 22-23

Night Training

Be ready for anything at any time.
—SEAL

New York City to Connecticut
11° to 9°
1400

It's the Christmas holiday! New York City is lit up and beautiful. If you have never been to New York during this time, it really is special. The streets are quiet and all the stores are shut down as people prepare to spend the day with loved ones celebrating.

Our family, which now includes SEAL, decides to head back up to Connecticut. I love the holidays, especially with all the winter elements. There's something in the air that just makes me feel festive. Regardless of religion or beliefs, for the most part everyone is in the spirit of giving. Even SEAL.

SEAL and I head out for a quick six-mile run in the mountains. It is a maintenance run at an 8:30 clip. Meaning

we are not getting better during this run, but we are not getting worse either. We are "maintaining our shit," he tells me.
When we get back home, I shower up and change.

I meet Sara in the family room. As she and I exchange
some Hannukah and Christmas gifts, SEAL comes into the
room holding something in his hands. He's protecting it like a
fullback would a football near the goal line.

"Your boy's got an inner toughness," SEAL says. "I
wanted to capture that in a gift," and he hands a present to
Lazer.

I'm wondering, Is it a toy truck? Blocks? Soccer ball?
Nope. It's a miniature camouflage outfit, complete with hat.
Real Army fatigues...a unique gift for a two-year-old!

Sara then gives SEAL a present from us. (She really
wanted to.) And right after he opens it, she asks him to try
it on. He politely declines. SEAL isn't big into receiving
gifts. Most humans like gifts, SEAL looks at gifts like they
are clutter. She asks again and he respectfully says, "Later."
By the third time my wife is no longer asking, she's insisting.
Even SEAL doesn't dare mess with her.

SEAL goes into the bedroom to change. But now he
doesn't want to come out. But after a minute or two, he reluctantly appears.

Out walks SEAL in a very nice casual dress shirt. Your
standard, light-blue button-down. It looks nice on him. But
judging from SEAL's expression, you'd think he's wearing a
straitjacket.

I hand Sara the gifts that I got her the other day at Barneys. She can tell by the size of the box that it's jewelry. She
opens it up and puts the necklace around her neck.

"I love it, sweetie. But what I really love is that you went out of your way for me. Love you."

A for effort!

1900

It's frigid and snowy. The family is feeling good. We're all together. A typical late December in the Itzler household might be a fire in the fireplace, some blankets, and a movie once Lazer goes to bed. I'd usually vote for something with a little bit of edge to it, but Sara would lobby and win for a romantic comedy.

"It's bedtime," Sara says to Lazer.

He's on the floor playing with SEAL. They've got action heroes and Matchbox cars and are saving the world. Somehow SEAL has created a realistic village made up of blocks and tanks attacking from all directions. SEAL is barking orders like it's a real-life raid. He's taking it way too seriously, but Lazer is actually interested and looks like he's enjoying himself. Which alarms me.

0200

It's 2:00 a.m. and snowing like crazy. The door to my bedroom is locked and I'm sleeping when I hear what sounds like someone trying to pick the lock of my door. The door handle is making noises like it's being pulled and tugged from the other side of the door. Then the sound I hear is like when a dog is scratching to get into the room while the handle is being pulled and tugged some more.

I get out of my bed to check. I put my ear to the door to hear what's going on, but now I don't hear anything. Silence. So I bend down and get on all fours to look under the door crack to see if I see anything. Sure enough, I see SEAL's sneakers by the door. I stand up and pull open the door and SEAL is standing right there.

"It's time," he says.

SEAL tells me the plan is to run four miles every four hours for forty-eight hours!

Twelve runs of four miles each *every four hours*! He calls it the 4/4/48.

Are you kidding me?

Apparently, he's not. In fact, we're going to train for it by

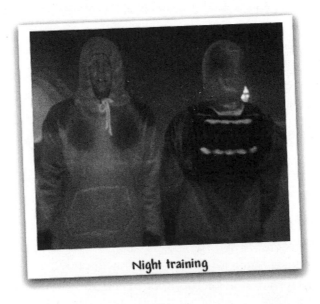

Night training

running 4.25 miles four times in twenty-four hours, or four runs every six hours.

I'm about to ask SEAL his logic behind this, but instead I just say, "Are you kidding me?"

0230

I open up my phone so I can get the light on it to shine and then I use it as a flashlight. I don't want to put the bedroom lights on because that might wake up Sara. She has been super cool about everything to date, but I'm not sure she would want me running in the snow at 2:00 a.m. in the mountains of Connecticut.

I go to my closet and quietly open up my drawers to get my gear. I feel like I'm sleepwalking, but I know that is wishful thinking. I layer up, tiptoe out of our bedroom, and head downstairs to the front door. SEAL is already outside.

I'm wearing a thermal, a hoodie, a hat, two pairs of gloves, and thermal pants. SEAL is in shorts, a hoodie, and gloves. It's freezing outside. Wet and freezing. We head out.

Every step feels like I'm about to fall off the earth. It's pitch black. I mean *pitch*. Five minutes into the run, SEAL turns to me and says, "Rough road ahead. Twenty meters."

Now, how could he possibly know that? I can't see one meter in front of me. In fact, I'm not sure I even know what a meter is. I mastered military time, but I'm not up on the metric system. Anyway, apparently, SEAL's eyesight isn't affected by darkness. It's like he has night vision without the night-vision goggles. He sees fine.

It's also bitter cold. My fingertips are completely numb. SEAL runs like he's in Anguilla, it's eighty degrees and sunny.

Meanwhile, the snow hits my frozen face like BB gun pellets. I'm squinting to see and closing my eyes for thirty seconds at a clip to keep the snow from pounding into my eyeballs. I'm no longer in the holiday spirit.

Soon we hit a patch of rough road. I say to myself, That must be how far twenty meters is. We move on.

We run 4.5 miles in exactly forty minutes. When we get home, we don't even turn the lights on. Our eyes are so adjusted to the dark that I can actually see fine in my pitch-dark house. Apparently SEAL's built in night-vision goggles have rubbed off on me.

I strip naked and put all of my clothing in the dryer. My skin has red blotches all over from the cold and I am freezing. I put on two sweatshirts and a ski hat and get into bed. Sara is sound asleep next to me.

Approximately four hours later...

My phone alarm goes off. I got about three hours of sleep. I get my clothes out of the dryer. If only they were still warm. SEAL is waiting at the front door. When we open the door, a bunch of snow falls into my foyer. It's twelve degrees outside.

We head out.

It's still as dark outside as when we got in from the last run, and it's still as cold and wet. It's like groundhog night. My muscles are super stiff from the cold (and the mileage), and my feet hurt when they hit the hard, snowy pavement. We do the same run as before in thirty-eight minutes. Brutal.

Four hours later...
19°

It's run number three in our twenty-four hours of runs every four hours. The hardest part so far has been the process of exerting myself, cooling down, and then having to start again. The restart is a bitch. SEAL throws me a bone and says if we do the loop in less than thirty-eight minutes, we don't have to run again in four hours. That's a bone I like!

Thus begins the great debate: Do we go out hard (the first mile is very tough with big elevation) or do we pace ourselves?

SEAL says, "Go hard."

"Let's go!" I say.

Out of a hundred runs on this mountain course, my fastest first mile *ever* is exactly 9:00. Trust me, this run is *hilly*. We do this one in 8:07! We are flying! I'm gasping for air. Literally. As we get to the top of the hill (1.1 miles) I feel like I'm cramping. I keep going and it gets worse. I can't run.

"Stop the clock for a second, something's off."

Groin pull?

It's so damn cold out I can't officially diagnose myself until we get home. We walk the one mile back. The sweat pours off of me. I guess SEAL was right, it's eighty and sunny, but with each step back, it feels like the temperature drops a degree. Then my body heat mixes with the cold and creates a thick, white vapor that rises from my skin. I'm a human chimney. After we get home and defrost, I confirm it. It is indeed my groin. I'm in abject pain. It's impossible to run.

"Push-ups instead," SEAL says.

We do ten sets of thirty (with a one-minute break in between). Drops of ice start to fall off my face as I go down and start the push-up routine.

"Is this the hardest forty-eight hours you've ever had?" SEAL asks.

"Physically, yeah," I say. "Then again, this is even harder than the Grant Hill shit."

"The basketball player?"

"Yeah," I say.

"You trained with him?"

"No."

"Then what the fuck are you talking about?"

One time Foot Locker hired me and my partner Kenny to do a national radio campaign. It was part of the work we were doing for our company Alphabet City. We were up against some other agencies, but we won the account because I promised them I could get Grant Hill to be in the commercial. Hill had been the NBA's Rookie of the Year and was a bona fide rising superstar. He was a big get. They wanted him and I promised we would get him.

"No problem," I said.

But, there was a problem—I didn't know Grant Hill.

After we signed Foot Locker to do the campaign, I learned Grant was making an appearance at a Foot Locker in Manhattan, so my plan was to approach him right at the event. All I needed to do was get Hill to say something like: "Hi, this is Grant Hill and I'm shopping at Foot Locker this holiday season," and then insert it into the radio spot. Then Foot Locker would give him a $500 gift certificate and I would be on my way.

Easy, right?

Except that I missed the event. I could go into a whole long explanation of what happened, but I'll save you the time. I just blew it. The next day the CEO of Foot Locker called me and asked if I got Grant Hill and I had to tell him no.

"You've got forty-eight hours," he said. "Or the deal's off."

I immediately got the NBA schedule and found out the Orlando Magic, Grant Hill's team, was playing the Hawks that night. I went straight to LaGuardia and headed for Atlanta. I got to the arena at 10:30 in the morning even though the game didn't tip-off until 7:30 at night. It was so early that I was able to walk right into the arena. Some marching band was rehearsing, and nobody questioned me because I was "with the band."

I knew that players typically showed up at 5:30 for a 7:30 game, so I had a lot of time to kill. I just walked around like I knew what I was doing. I just tried to look busy.

Though it seemed like forever, eventually some of the Orlando Magic began to show up. I stood at a payphone and pretended to make a call as I waited for Grant. And then I saw my mark. I walked right up to him as he came through the player entrance.

"Hey, Grant, it's Jesse from Foot Locker. I flew down and I'm here to get the audio clip I was supposed to get on Saturday," I said. "You ready now?"

"What audio clip?"

"Right. The audio clip from the Foot Locker event."

"Okay, let's talk about it after the game," he said, walking past me.

"No, no," I said. "I have to get it now and get back on the plane."

He kept walking into the locker room, so I leaned over and pulled his ear close to my mouth. "Grant, look into my eyes. I'm going to lose my job if I don't get this done. I can't go home without this. I flew down here on my own dime today to get this. I don't know what it is, but they need it. The CEO sent me."

Maybe he saw the genuine fear in my eyes or heard it in my plea. Whatever the case, he obliged.

"Okay," he said. "Follow me."

So I walked into the locker room with all of the players goofing off and starting to get ready for the game. I pull out my handheld recorder and hand him a script. BUT...it's too loud in the locker room, so I take him into the bathroom stall and close the door.

I hand Grant the script again and push record.

"Hey, this is Grant Hill, and this holiday season you can find me at Foot Locker. Foot Locker has got you covered."

Halfway through the third line he said, "Who are you again? And what is this being used for?"

"Grant, I've been on the phone with your agent all day. This is part of the Foot Locker package you did. They're running a holiday promotion." I was just throwing words at him. "It's the audio part." I was hoping he might pick up some buzzwords and think that I actually was supposed to be there.

"Okay, fine," he said, and he finished it and then I ran out.

As soon as I got out of the arena, I headed back to the airport and called Kenny from another payphone and played him the recording. The next day it was on national radio.

"That's some funny shit," Seal says without cracking a smile.

"Do you want to hear about the big red chicken now?"

"No."

3:00 p.m.

SEAL takes me down to the gym to do some push-ups. Our Connecticut house has a gym on the bottom floor. Adjacent to the gym is a steam room and a sauna. It's like a mini training facility, and I love hanging out down there.

I bought this house seven years ago and gutted the entire place right after the closing. At the time I was building Marquis Jet, and I wanted a place where I could entertain customers. One of the most important things I told the decorator was that I wanted a steam room that you never want to leave. Yeah, I picked out colors and approved floor plans, but I really only cared about the steam room. This gym and spa area are my personal retreat.

We do twenty sets of twenty push-ups with a one-minute break in between each set. Let me repeat...twenty sets of twenty push-ups!!! The first ten are actually fairly easy. But the second half starts to get the better of me. I push my way through it and get to the final set. I'm *jacked-up* sore.

"Finish up. GET THIS SHIT DONE, FUCKER."

I do. I have to hold a plank position in between reps for about twenty seconds on each of the last twenty push-ups, but I get it done.

That's seven hundred so far today including the three hundred we did earlier.

SEAL begs me to do three hundred more to get to a thousand push-ups. He begs me!

"I physically can't," I say.

And I mean it. I can't do one more push-up. I can't even hold a downward dog pose. I head upstairs with my arms dangling by my sides.

We call it a day and I relax on my couch. I grab the *Sports Business Journal* and get caught up on recent transactions. The few hours of downtime are like a vacation, and I'm feeling cozy.

Workout totals: 16.1 miles and 700 push-ups

DAY 24

Whiteout

The tougher the conditions, the more I like my odds.
—SEAL

Connecticut

5°

0600

We wake up to blizzard conditions. Sixteen inches of snow with 30-mph winds and –7 degrees with wind chill. Miraculously my groin feels better. Maybe it was just a cramp?

Repeatedly scrolling across the bottom of my television screen is an "EXTREME WEATHER WARNING." The local news in Connecticut is advising everyone to "STAY INSIDE UNLESS IT'S AN EMERGENCY."

"This is fucking perfect," SEAL says.

I guess he considers this an emergency.

He stares at the TV, bobbing his head like he's listening to Jay Z, only he's not wearing any headphones.

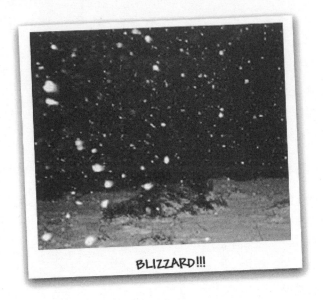

BLIZZARD!!!

Finally he says, "We gotta head out."

We run 3.5 miles in the mountains.

SEAL decides to wear the fifty-pound weight vest. He is *out of his mind*. I can't explain how hard this run is...in these conditions...with a fifty-pound weight vest on. When we get home, I think I'm frostbitten. My shirt is so cold and wet it hurts to take it off. In fact, my shirt is actually frozen. When I manage to get it off, it sits upright in my chair.

We do 144 push-ups, plus an extra ten for good measure.

2:00 p.m.

Sara goes outside to get the mail. The mailbox is at the end of our driveway, about fifty yards away once you walk out of the front door. The only obstacle or "threat" between our front door and getting our mail is the grass, which is covered by snow. The danger would be that someone slips on a patch of ice. What I mean is…getting the mail is not a high-wire act. It's not something on our radar as far as a thing to worry about.

Sara returns holding three envelopes and a fashion catalog. She begins to open the catalog.

SEAL is livid.

"Sara, you need to mix up your pattern."

"Pattern?"

"Yeah, your pattern. PATTERN. The time you get the mail. That's your pattern. It's the same every day. It's predictable."

"I get the mail after lunch," she says. "That's the most convenient time."

"Why after lunch?" SEAL asks baffled. "That seems common."

"Because that's when the mailman comes," she replies. "He delivers the mail after lunch."

"Exactly. You know that. And I know that. The mailman most definitely knows that. So I bet EVERYONE knows that. For sure your neighbors know that."

"But I'm just getting the mail…at my house…on our property," she says.

"Just do me a favor. Change up the pickup time. Go an hour or so later tomorrow. Break the pattern, Sara. Break the pattern."

2100

Sara and I have dinner before we put Lazer down for bed. Nothing fancy, just some veggie burgers and salad that we whipped up. Shortly after we get Lazer to sleep, we get into bed together to watch some TV. I'm fading into sleep land but can sense that Sara is still up and watching CNN.

At around 9:00 p.m. I feel Sara getting out of bed. She is doing it in a way not to wake me, but I'm slowly learning to be on alert. I'm awake.

"Where you going, sweetie?" I ask.

"I hear something in the basement. It sounds like our generator has kicked in."

"What are you talking about?"

Sara heads down before I can ask another question to check out the noise.

About eight minutes later Sara returns. She crawls back into bed and tells me, "No biggie." SEAL is on the stationary bike. He wants to "get some mileage in" and didn't want to "ride in the snow."

The next morning, we wake up at 7:00 a.m. and the generator sound is *still* making the same noise. This time I head downstairs. As I get closer I can hear the noise coming from the gym, and music is playing in the background. I open the door to the gym and a wave of hot air attacks me. It's like someone is holding a hair dryer on high and pointing it at my face. The room feels like a sauna and the windows are all fogged up. Straight ahead I see SEAL on the stationary bike with his shirt off and puddles of sweat on the floor. He doesn't look up. Clearly he knows I'm there, but he does *not* say a word. Not even a hello or good morning. He doesn't look happy—shocker, I know. He keeps riding.

He rode the entire night. Ten hours straight.

Workout totals: 3.5 miles and 154 push-ups

DAY 25

Get Your Balls Wet

Fear is one of the best motivators.
Anger is the other.
—SEAL

Connecticut
5°
0930

SEAL takes me on a five-mile run up Wanzer Hill. Wanzer
Hill is the main road in my development, and it's so steep
it's almost vertical. There should be double black diamonds
on the street sign. Cars can't get up it in good weather.
Other hills don't even want to be in the same neighborhood
as Wanzer Hill, it's that intimidating. Plus, there's snow and
black ice everywhere, making the run slower/harder/colder.

Didn't SEAL just ride a bike all night? WTF! He didn't
stop.

When we get home after the run, I complain that the

tendon in my foot is killing me (recurring basketball injury) and my foot is swollen. Really swollen.

"I got a solution. Let's go into the lake and freeze your foot," SEAL says.

"Go into the lake? The lake's frozen."

"I'm not playing. Let's go," he says.

I know this is the dumbest idea ever, but there is something about it I like. I get excited. I've always wondered how cold the water under the top layer of ice in a frozen lake is. We run down the hill from my house to the lake in two feet of snow. I am in sneakers, socks, shorts, and a sweatshirt. It's about three hundred yards at a steady decline. I stumble twice and face-plant before I reach the bottom. SEAL descends flawlessly and effortlessly. When we arrive, he immediately takes off his shoes and finds a hole in the ice big enough to fit him.

And *jumps in*! The lake is frozen but not completely. Parts of the lake by the shore have thin patches of ice.

"Hold on to the floating ice," he says.

I swear this happened.

I crawl onto the frozen lake and inch my way toward the hole where SEAL jumped in.

"GET THE FUCK IN, MOTHERFUCKER. GET THE FUCK IN!"

He's lost his mind.

"NO. I can't. I'm sorry. I can't."

"Get the fuck in, motherfucker. Get the fuck in," he says again. His lips are blue. "You fucking pussy, Itzler, get the fuck in!"

I take off my shoes. I take off my socks. This is insane.

"Get in. Balls deep. GET IN, ITZLER."

I jump in up to my knees. It feels like someone is sawing off my legs. Or maybe it feels like I wish someone would saw off my legs.

"DEEPER," he yells. I inch my way deeper, up to my waist.

Then, all of a sudden, his expression changes. It's no longer taut with anger. Now it's furrowed and worried.

"We got five minutes till frostbite. GET OUT NOW!"

What?!

"Don't touch your skin to the ice as you get out, it'll stick," he yells.

"*What?*"

"Like that motherfucker in *Christmas Story*. Grab your sneakers and use them as gloves, climb out of the hole in the ice, and crawl across the ice with your BARE FEET sticking up," he yells.

It takes two minutes to get to land. My mind is counting down like MacGyver. We have about three minutes left until frostbite. We run up the hill toward my house, with shoes off, barefoot in the snow.

SEAL's yelling again, "WE HAVE TWO MINUTES… RUN."

Halfway up the hill, my body is fueled by fear. There isn't a coherent thought in my head other than to get up this hill. My toes are going to fall off. I can't feel one thing from my knees down. With each stride I take I feel like my legs could shatter like an antique teacup hitting the floor. This is bad.

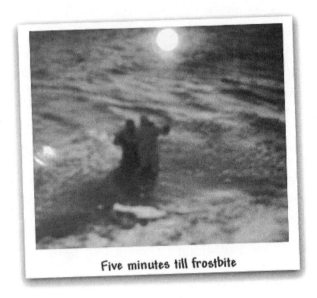

Five minutes till frostbite

Finally we reach the top. We go inside, peel off our wet clothing, dry off with towels and coats and anything we can grab.

Sara stands there, and I don't think I've ever seen her so angry. "That's the dumbest thing I've ever seen!" she yells.

"I'm sorry," I say.

"Sorry? You're a dad! Everyone knows not to go near ice on a *frozen lake.*"

She turns to SEAL. "And you!" she says to him. "You ought to be ashamed of yourself. Tell me what the medical benefit of jumping into a frozen lake is."

"There is none, Sara! This is what your husband SIGNED UP FOR!!! There's no benefit."

Fifteen minutes later...

SEAL comes and finds me and says, "We got to capitalize on this shit. We got to capitalize on this adrenaline."

What?

We do fifteen sets of fifteen push-ups on the minute (225 push-ups). The entire time I'm thinking to myself, Nobody would ever believe this. Nobody. But I'm so far into it I am now embracing the challenges. It's like I'm over the hump and I can't help but feel a little proud.

Twenty minutes later...

SEAL comes into my bedroom. I'm sitting with my feet elevated to ease my swollen ankle. "We only have four days left. We need to push our limits. Your work isn't done. You aren't ready to go back to the real world," SEAL says.

I pause and then realize...he's right. My life with SEAL isn't the real world. Then I think about him leaving. There's going to be a huge hole. These past twenty-five days have been unlike any other in my life. I didn't think this was possible, but I'm going to miss him. I'm going to miss the insanity. I'm going to miss the pain. I'm going to miss having him in charge.

"Let's make tacos tonight for dinner," I say.

"Tacos? Fuck the tacos," he says. "We're going to go into the steam room."

"The steam room?"

"Yeah, the fucking steam room. Setting that bitch at one hundred twenty-five degrees and we're in there for thirty minutes. No dumping water on our heads, no talking (obviously), and only twelve ounces of drinking water allowed in. I'm going to test your WILL."

SEAL sets the temp dial for 125 and we wait twenty minutes until it is properly heated. We strip to our undies and go in. To maximize the effect, SEAL tells me to sit on my hands and keep my arms locked straight. That will force our backs to be straight and our heads to be closer to the ceiling of the steam.

"Heat rises," he says.

NO KIDDING!

By keeping our heads up, we will get "maximum exposure," he repeats.

So, we go in.

Five minutes...okay.

Ten minutes...okay.

Twelve minutes...I drink all twelve ounces of water.

Fifteen minutes... okay.

Twenty minutes...Not so okay.

I hear a hissing sound.

It's hard for me to see with my eyeballs sweating.

I hope the hissing isn't coming out of me.

My heart rate is up and pounding. My skin looks like boiled chicken.

I'm overheating.

I'm nauseous.

SEAL sits in the opposite corner of the steam room, and I can barely make him out. I hear him whistling, and it is driving me mad. It sounds like a Beach Boys song. It can't be.

I'm hallucinating. *Only nine more minutes*, I tell myself. But it's not working. I try to think about baseball: Jeter's baseball average; Jason Kipnis's fielding percentage; Mariano Rivera's WHIP.

I'M LOSING MY MIND!

Now I know how a Hot Pocket feels inside a microwave.

One, two, three, four... I start counting to one hundred in my head. *Eleven, twelve, thirteen*...

I'm drifting into Faint City.

"I don't think I can do it," I say, finally breaking the twenty-one minutes of silence. "I'm sorry."

I don't wait for him to respond. I leap up and thrust open the door, almost breaking the glass.

SEAL follows me out, steam pouring into the room as the door stays open.

"Okay. Thirty-second rest and then back in."

I don't move. He looks closer.

"Whoa," he says, looking down at me crouched against the wall. "You don't look so good."

He looks blurry and his face is distorted like in a fun house mirror.

"Goarblogger rasootoootle," I respond.

"Man, we need to ABORT," he says.

Abort?

I sit in the chair outside my steam room for what feels like a day. Alone. SEAL does not come to check on me. My head is pounding. After thirty-five minutes, I finally begin to cool down. My heart rate is at 119. I'm sweating like I am in the desert in August. I down five Zicos, and it takes ninety minutes before I begin to feel remotely human.

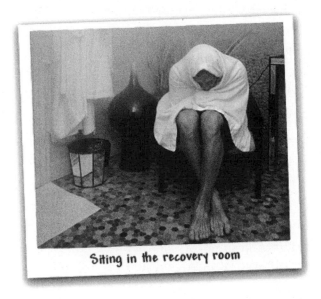

Siting in the recovery room

Two hours later...

I have relocated to my bedroom and SEAL comes in. I'm under the covers watching CNN. He asks if I'm better.

"A little," I say.

"Good. Let's go."

Let's go?

"You don't even know what suffering is, motherfucker," he says with a look like he means it. He's right. I've lived a sheltered life.

He tells me to do a slow jog by myself outside "to loosen up my joints." (The ones that were fused together in the steam room or the ones that were frozen together in the lake?) He wants me to "understand myself better." He wants me to "feel the isolation." I'm not sure where he is going with this. In fact, I don't know what the hell he is talking about.

But I go outside.

Alone.

Before I leave, he hands me a flashlight because it is starting to get dark so early now. "Watch the black ice," he says.

"Thanks."

I do a 4.5-mile slow jog. When I come home, SEAL is waiting at the door. He is literally sitting outside by my front door in the snow eating a fucking apple.

"Nice work. You need that personal mind frame," he says. I still have no idea what he is talking about.

"Now get your strength up and do a hundred push-ups before you can come in the house. That's ten every thirty seconds. I'm not fucking around, man, this isn't sleep-away camp in upstate Fuckville."

Again, what?

But I get down and start to knock out the push-ups. SEAL disqualifies my first one.

"Start over. Your nose needs to touch the snow. We are past the make-believe shit."

2000

Fuck tacos is right. I heat up two veggie burgers. I'm obsessed with the MorningStar Grillers Prime and tonight I feel like I can eat the whole box. As soon as the microwave beeps indicating my meal is ready, in comes SEAL.

"You got a choice: Eat first and do 250 push-ups *or* eat after and choose to do what's behind curtain number two."

All of a sudden he is Bob Barker? I don't even ask a single question, I just say, "Give me door number two."

Well...*more push-ups.* We do twelve, then eight, then six, then four push-ups on the fifteen-second mark, followed by sit-ups, where we do as many as we can for sixty seconds. We rest one minute, then repeat for thirty minutes.

I'm a beaten man.

> **Workout totals: 9.5 miles, 775 push-ups, 125 sit-ups, 21-minute steam, frozen lake**

DAY 26

Primary Target

Know what's important to you and protect it
at all costs.
—SEAL

Connecticut
29°
0800

I'm fully recovered from the steam room incident. We're still
in Connecticut, and SEAL and I head out for the 4.5-mile
mountain loop near my house. I'm breathing just through my
nose. It feels like I'm flying. I check my time: 35:17. That's
three minutes faster than my previous personal best. Course
record for me! I'm feeling good.

We get home, shower, and meet in the den. I turn the
TV on.

Getting SEAL to watch television can be difficult. The
only thing I've seen him sit still for is sports. There are a few
college football bowl games on today so I'm hoping he won't

ask me to wear the fifty-pound weight vest in the second and fourth quarters. He seems fairly content on the couch. I wonder if he's thinking about leaving. The thought has been on my mind the last couple of days. At first, to be honest, I couldn't wait for the month to be over. But he's starting to grow on me. I appreciate his concern for my family's safety. It makes me wonder...

"Say, SEAL," I say. "What would you do if there was an intruder in the house?"

Slowly SEAL turns and looks at me. He holds me with an even, unemotional stare. Then he turns back to the TV without answering my question.

"No, really," I say. "What would you do?"

He shakes his head slowly.

"I think you know what I'd do," he says to the TV.

"Tell me."

"I would protect the primary."

"What's the primary?"

"That's the million-dollar question," he says. "What is your primary, Jesse? What would hurt you the most to lose? This big-screen TV? Those gold record awards you own? Jewelry? Cash? What do you hold most dear?"

"No," I say. "None of that."

"Well?" he asks.

"My wife and my son."

"Exactly, Jesse," he says. "They're your primary, and as long as I'm in this house they're my primary too. You asked me what I would do. I would protect my primary at any cost. And unfortunately for you, you're my third option."

At that moment I realize that despite all the time I have

spent with SEAL, he has always had an eye on Sara and Lazer. The plumber, the white van, the waiter...it's all been about protecting "us." Sure we have been training, but there is more to our relationship now. We have "primaries" to look after.

2100

I tell SEAL that I have to spend a few hours "closing the books" for the year, and I beg him not to interrupt me. He agrees.

"Go ahead and handle your shit, man."

I pull out all my notes and "to do" lists from this past year and take some personal inventory. I also make my annual donations and send out our holiday cards. It feels good to close out the year.

Once I come out from my office, he tells me, "We gotta get one in."

We go out for a five-mile run at top speed. I push, my body responds. Holy shit, I feel fit. Almost immortal. I feel up for anything! I think this is starting to pay off!

Workout totals: 9.5 miles

DAY 27

1,000 Push-ups

I don't celebrate victories but I learn from failures.
—SEAL

Connecticut
12°
0800

SEAL says "Today is goal day. Today all your hard work pays off. We are going to see if you can do one thousand push-ups."

I start the day off with ten quick sets of ten push-ups. We take a thirty-second rest in between sets. Feeling good. I rest.

Total: 100 push-ups

Two hours later...

First 1–18 push-ups and then one set of twenty-nine (8:58). Maybe I'm relying on muscle memory as I have done this already, but still feeling good. Rest again.

Total: 200 push-ups.

One hour later...

1–18 push-ups and then one set of twenty-nine (8:30). Now it's a struggle. I'm grinding these out. The last fifty I have to hold a plank position for a few seconds before I go down and up.

    Total: 200 push-ups.

Three hours later...

1–18 push-ups and then one set of twenty-nine (8:30). Now I am getting into the REALLY HARD territory. I'm taking long breaks in between each push-up group. But, I'm doing it. My triceps are on FIRE.

    Total: 200 push-ups.

1600

25, 25, 25, 25–1–18, 15, 14. These are BRUTAL. My arms are shaking like a leaf. My triceps feel like they have pins in them. It's a feeling I have never had before and I'm actually a bit concerned. SEAL tells me to "push through." My arms are trembling.

    "Push through it," he yells.

    I have to take a two-minute break before I complete the set of fifteen. Then I need a five-minute break before I can complete the last fourteen. But, once I'm close...there is no giving up!

Total: 300 push-ups.

In case you didn't count 'em, that's one thousand.

One thousand push-ups!

In one day. *Holy shit!* I take a seat on my couch by the steam room and smile. For the first time during this whole process, I'm truly proud of myself. Not because I did a thousand but because I stuck with the journey. I think back to the first day SEAL was here and the first set of push-ups we did. This proves to me that if you push the body, the body will respond.

1900

My body is inflated from all the push-ups. I feel like I'm wearing a wetsuit and someone has pumped air into it. I'm jacked up. But to SEAL, victories are short-lived. He tells me he never celebrates an accomplishment. Once his goal is done, it's time for his next goal. Our work is not done. It's time for our next goal.

SEAL and I head out for a 3.5-mile run.

When we get home, SEAL tells me to "get some shut-eye" and that "I earned it." I'm not sure, but I think that's a compliment. He is actually proud of me too. I go into my room and throw on ESPN to watch some Bowl highlights. SEAL heads to his room. He goes and continues to do twenty-five push-ups every ten minutes, 4:30 until midnight. He does twenty-five hundred for the day. *Superhuman.*

With fitness there's never a finish line. You can always do better. For me personally, I guess I probably have thirty or forty years left on earth. And how many of those am I going to be young enough and healthy enough to do things? I want to experience the best stuff I can. I've never jumped off a cliff—I should just jump off a cliff because I'm only here once. That's how I approach things now. That's how I feel about things. That's how I live my life.

A thousand push-ups is something I could never have imagined doing. It just shows that repetition and consistency equal results.

Workout totals: 3.5 miles and 1,000 push-ups!

DAY 28

Up the Ante

If you don't challenge yourself, you don't know
yourself.
—SEAL

Connecticut
17°
0700

This morning we go for an 8.5-mile run up Leach Hollow
Road and back. Getting to Leach Hollow Road is not easy.
My friend Fish calls it "the Big Boy Run." It's a freak show.
Crazy hills, grueling course, and 8.5 miles is a good run
no matter how you slice it. I've run this course with many
friends, and only a select few have been able to complete it.

Anyway, I run it in 1:17:41 (an 8:57 average), with nega-
tive splits, which means clocking a better time the second
half of the run than the first. I'm two minutes faster on the
way back and I'm feeling psyched.

When we get home, the real fun begins.

"We have to up the ante," SEAL says.

"The lake?" I ask.

SEAL nods.

I begin to nod with him.

We stand there both understanding the mission and nodding together.

One little problem. This time there are no holes in the lake. It's frozen solid—six inches thick. There are even kids playing hockey on it.

"I have a plan," SEAL says.

"If you two knuckleheads even think about going through the ice again," Sara says, "don't bother coming back inside. It's frozen solid."

It's like my wife has a crystal ball or something. I didn't even see her standing there. She knows the nod. But I know Sara has a conference call later. So we wait.

When SEAL is sure my wife isn't watching, he sneaks down to the lake, grabs a boulder, and starts banging on the ice. And when I say boulder, I mean boulder, like from *The Flintstones*. This thing is huge, and SEAL has to bend down and lift with his legs and hold it with both hands before he can hoist it up. I look over at the kids skating and the game comes to an ice-spraying hockey stop. They are all watching SEAL.

SEAL pounds away: Boom-crackle crackle...Again... Boom-crackle crackle...Again...Boom-crackle crackle...

The hockey players head to solid ground.

The ice breaks. I think somewhere in SEAL's inner ear there's a tiny orchestra playing the theme song from *Rocky*. It's like he's at the top of the stairs of the Philadelphia

Museum of Art and he raises his arms in a victory pose. He gives a primal scream of "YESSSS!"

Socks off, shirt off...he's in!!!!

I start to hear the *Rocky* theme too.

I can do this...socks off, shirt off, I'm in!!!!

We repeat this twice and sprint up to my house to get warm.

I'm still freezing but feel: AMAZING!

Sara stands in the doorway. She glares at me but doesn't say a word. She gives the same stern look to SEAL. I feel like I'm seven. SEAL, who doesn't raise his eyes, looks like he's five.

My son is staring at my feet and looking puzzled. They have a reddish purple tint to them.

And SEAL...now he's on the TREADMILL!

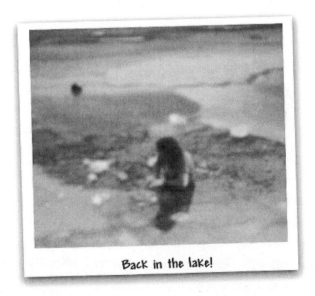

Back in the lake!

We're in the penalty box for about half the day. Sara wasn't really that mad, at least not at our houseguest. It's like she wanted to be mad, but she couldn't. Maybe it's because she knows all of this is coming to an end or perhaps she knows I'll probably never do this again. It's not safe.

5:00 p.m. . . . thirty minutes before dinner

We do ten push-ups on the thirty-second hand for ten sets (every five minutes).

That's a hundred total.

Then it's 1–10, 10–1, and three sets of thirty.

Another three hundred down!

8:00 p.m.

I'm in the bedroom with Sara, packing. We're going to Atlanta tomorrow but just staying overnight.

"What day is SEAL leaving again?" Sara asks.

"In two days," I say. "He'll come to Atlanta and then spend New Year's with us back here in Connecticut, but he's going home from there."

"I'm going to miss him," she says.

Sara had already told me that SEAL was the best houseguest we've ever had. She didn't have to tell him how to do anything or where anything was. He didn't need any instructions: He was spotless, thoughtful, and polite. But when SEAL really won her over is when Sara's grandmother, Nannie, stopped by one day in Atlanta. Nannie's right out of *The Andy Griffith Show*. SEAL was a total gentleman and did everything for her: carried her bags, made her breakfast, and walked with her on his arm. She adored him. When Nannie was around, I think she was SEAL's primary! Nannie kept referring to SEAL as "that nice young man." She would say, "Jesse, that nice young man…that friend of yours is just darling."

Sara seems to be very intently folding a blouse.

"I've been thinking," she says after a moment or two. "We should try and get SEAL to stay a bit longer."

As I'm looking at my wife packing it makes me realize what a difference a month can make. I know SEAL infinitely better than I did when he first showed up, but I still don't know him know him. But I think that's by design.

Sara snaps me back to present day with the toss of a diaper. I guess she knows something I don't. I catch the diaper and am about to make my way to Lazer when she looks at me.

"I've been giving it some thought. And I think I'd like to start a workout routine with SEAL too."

"Okay, sweetie. If that's what you really want, then ask him."

I'm acting cool, but I'm *psyched*!!!

"Just don't expect me to jump in the frozen lake," she says.

Workout totals: 8.5 miles, 300 push-ups, frozen lake

DAY 29

Sloppy Seconds

I don't stop when I'm tired. I stop when I'm done.
—SEAL

Connecticut to Atlanta
36° to 88°
0900

We're leaving for a day trip to Atlanta this afternoon to do another check on the house, but first we head out on a 10.6-mile run in the rain and slush. It's warmed up a bit and the roads are sloppy.

"We gotta get one good one in before the flight," SEAL says.

The run is from my house to a diner on Route 22. I have no idea what the name of the diner is, but it is the *only* diner near us. I also know that when we drive up to the house from New York City, it's a marker for us. When we get to the diner, it's still a fifteen-minute drive. So the run is not going to be fun.

As predicted, it's lonely, miserable, hilly, and tough. I tell Sara we will be about an hour and a half and that we are running to the diner.

"You are going to run to the diner that we order takeout from? You *got to be kidding me.*"

"I kid you not," I reply.

"Can you pick me up some—" she says with a laugh.

SEAL must not have taken his patience pill when he took his handful of vitamins today because as soon as we start the run, he takes off. Every few straightaways he becomes visible for the first few miles, but then he completely disappears. He beats me there by eighteen minutes.

Time: 1:36:00.

Sara jumps in the car and picks us up at the diner ninety-five minutes after we leave the house.

Ninety minutes later...

It's noon. "We have to get to the airport in a few hours," I say to SEAL. "Sara will kill us if we are late."

Two minutes later he has me on the treadmill walking twenty minutes on a fifteen-degree incline at 3.6 pace.

"We'll get there," SEAL says.

Next it's three pull-ups every forty-five seconds for the next ten minutes.

"We gotta go."

"Relax."

We do ten push-ups on the thirty-second mark for another ten minutes.

Right before the last set SEAL says, "We clocked out.
Let's go."

> **Workout totals: 10.6 miles, 20 minutes on
> treadmill on incline of 15, 100 push-ups,
> 30 pull-ups**

The Skinheads

I don't like assholes and I don't like bullies.
—SEAL

The weather in Atlanta is fantastic. The hot Georgia sun is pumping out punishing heat rays. I'm sitting alone at the pool in my backyard reading the paper when our cleaning lady approaches. She's flustered. Her English is good, but sometimes the words are hard for her to find.

"You come, Mr. Jesse," she says. "I concern. Two guys in front yard ask for owner. Something no right, Mr. Jesse."

So I throw on a shirt and go out front.

Sure enough, there are two guys, approximately twenty years old, in white T-shirts and jeans, and they're climbing over our small hedges and approaching the front door. Both are heavily tatted up. Both have shaved heads. Both reek of marijuana.

She's correct, "Something no right."

It's mostly a mix of doctors, lawyers, and young professionals who live in our Atlanta community. People go out for jogs in the neighborhood or ride expensive mountain bikes around the cul-de-sac. And everybody smiles.

From the street you can see our house quite clearly. Nothing spectacular. It has a well-groomed yard, better-than-average-size driveway, and a decent-size house. While we do have some surveillance cameras around the exterior, you'd have to look closely to notice them.

"Can I help you guys?" I say in my most laid-back voice.

"Sure can," says Skinhead Number One. "Can you tell me who the owner of this house is?"

"Well, what exactly do you guys need?"

"We just moved into the neighborhood, son," he says.

The guy calls me "son" and I'm at least twenty years older than him.

"We want to meet a thousand neighbors. Each and every one of 'em. If we do, we get points for college."

Number One smiles and shows me some bullshit pad on a clipboard.

"We already met Usher today. You know where Usher lives, dude? Well, we seen 'em."

I know Usher doesn't live anywhere near me. I really think these guys are casing out my house.

HOLY SHIT!

"Sorry, guys. I don't live here. I'm only a guest," I lie.

"Well then, can you get your daddy or the queen bee? We need to meet the actual owner," Number Two says.

He looks like a number two.

Did this guy really just tell me to get my daddy?

"You want me to get my dad?"

"Yeah! Or go get the queen bee." Number One laughs. "Just get someone in the house that lives here."

"No problem," I say. "Hang tight."

I walk into the kitchen. SEAL is making one of his military-grade shakes.

"We have a situation," I say, looking out through the window that faces the front lawn.

SEAL follows my stare. A smile spreads across his face

as he looks through the window. The skinheads start to leave as if they sense something isn't right. SEAL calmly finishes drinking his shake.

"Showtime," he says.

Twenty minutes later SEAL is back walking through the front door. He has his iPhone in his hand. He shows me a close-up photo of Number Two. His face is as red as his neck and his cheeks are puffed up like a blowfish. His eyes are stretched with fear.

"This him?" SEAL asks.

In the photo you can see SEAL's hand wrapped around the guy's neck. It reminds me of when Darth Vader picks the guy up by his neck in *Star Wars*.

"Yes! That's him."

SEAL puts the phone in his pocket and walks over to the sink. He takes the glass from which he was drinking the shake and washes it.

"Well?"

"I explained to them I was the homeowner and that I don't care for motherfuckers like them on my property and that if they ever came back, I would make sure they never walked again."

SEAL puts the glass back in the cupboard. "I really don't think they'll be back."

Resolutions

I don't want what you guys have.

—SEAL

It's the last day of the year. Most people make resolutions on New Year's Eve, and I finished mine on the plane back to Connecticut this a.m.

Sara and I are having a bunch of our friends up to the house for dinner. We'll go around the table and everybody will say their goals for the coming year before dessert. I pretty much have what I'm going to say in my head. It's more like bullet points in my head. I'm a big fan of winging it (obviously).

The whole "Wonderful Wednesday" clan is coming. A few years ago, we made it an annual thing that we would get together for New Year's up at the Connecticut house. Sara calls us the SuperFriends because we also like to run marathons and other races together. There's a lot of truth to the "super" part. I've met, worked, and hung around a lot of people over my years. But the friends I have now are friends for life. These are the guys and girls I want to be in a foxhole with.

The day and night goes like this: We all go for a nine-mile run up Wanzer Hill and then have dinner, wine, whatever, and everyone sleeps over.

During dinner the conversation shifts to the resolutions. I'm curious about what SEAL will say if he takes a turn. In fact, I think everybody here is wondering what SEAL will say, if anything. One friend wants to quit her job and start her own business. Another has decided he wants to move to California's Wine Country. When it's SEAL's turn the whole table quiets.

"I don't want the same shit you guys want. I'm not looking for anything else. I'm going to do the same shit I've been doing," he says, "only I'm going to do it better."

SEAL excuses himself and stands. He then goes downstairs to ride the stationary bike in the basement. When he returns later my friends start to ask him questions. They're drawn to him. A big circle has formed around SEAL in the living room. He is still sweating from the ride, but he has placed a towel on his lap to catch any dripping sweat that could potentially end up on our carpet. The alcohol has loosened everyone up a bit. He looks at us all. His armor has come down. It's as though he's sorry for coming on so strong at the dinner table.

"I just think you don't give your lives enough credit," he says softly.

DAY 30

Last Run

If you can see yourself doing something, you can do
it. If you can't see yourself doing something, usually
you can't achieve it.
—SEAL

New York City
40°
1230

It's after lunchtime and we just drove back to New York City.
SEAL gave me the morning off. I'm in the kitchen cleaning
up. Sara and SEAL are in the living room. Then I see my
wife in the doorway.

"How'd it go with asking SEAL to stay and train you?" I ask.

"He can only stay one more day," Sara says. "He's leaving
tomorrow."

My wife can be a very convincing woman. I'm surprised.
"Did he say why?"

"Business."

"Business?"

Sara shrugs.

"That's it?"

"That's it."

I'm both disappointed he's not staying and bursting with curiosity. I know better than to ask him though. Anyhow, I like the image I conjure of SEAL pulling off a midnight hostage rescue in Syria or something.

"Oh, he did say he'd come back to train me," Sara says.

"Really?"

"Yes, provided I do everything he says and *nothing* is off limits."

Just that moment, SEAL walks into the kitchen. He's wearing the biggest smile I've ever seen him wear.

"What's for dinner tonight?" Seal asks. "A big red chicken?" He cackles like it's the funniest thing anyone has ever said. We head out to Central Park for the 6.1-mile loop. It will be our last run.

My first run with SEAL in New York was thirty days ago. We ran the exact same loop. We did it in 56:04 (a 9:20-mile pace). After one month with SEAL training me, I'm running a 7:50 pace per mile.

As usual, we don't talk on the run, even though it was to be our last. There was no final test, no congratulatory conversation, nothing. Like two running partners who run every day. There wasn't anything unusual about the evening either. We had dinner together in the apartment. SEAL played with Lazer. Sara chatted with him. Although she tried not to show it, I could tell she was genuinely sad our time with SEAL was coming to a close. So was I.

Today's splits:

Mile 1: 8:02
Mile 2: 7:56
Mile 3: 7:26
Mile 4: 7:45
Mile 5: 7:43
Mile 6: 7:32
Total: 46:34 (average of 7:45)

Pre-SEAL I sometimes would be on the couch and not want to do whatever needed to be done and I'd be like "Fuck it," and blow it off. Procrastinate.

I don't think like that anymore. Just get off the couch and do it is what I remind myself. SEAL would never say, "Fuck it." He'd get off the couch and do it. Regardless of the time, the temperature, or how tired he was. I absorbed some of that just-get-it-done and there-are-no-excuses attitude. I'm grateful for that.

My perspective on time has changed too. I got so much more done when SEAL was here. I was much more efficient. Now if I have to drive a few hours in the car to get somewhere, I do not get frustrated. Rather, I think about how lucky I am to be sitting in a warm and comfortable environment. It's weird, maybe I became more present or maybe I'm more appreciative, but whatever it is, I view time differently. Maybe it is a newfound patience or maturity.

My will to not stop or quit has also changed...both in training and at work.

SEAL has an I-don't-give-a-shit attitude that really

makes him different. He's an African-American Navy SEAL, of which there aren't many, an African-American who competes in endurance sports that are dominated by Caucasians. He doesn't give a shit. SEAL does what SEAL wants to do. He doesn't live the way everyone tells him he's supposed to live. And he does it with purpose. I admire him for that. His normal has been abnormal. We have that in common.

The first day SEAL came to move in, he told me I needed to control my mind. I thought it was just a saying or a throwaway comment, but I think there might be more truth to it than I originally thought. Our minds sometimes tell us little lies about ourselves, and we believe them. We think we can't do this or that. It's not true.

I've never had a real résumé. I've always believed in a life résumé. I take a look at SEAL, who's writing in his logbook. He just wants to get better tomorrow. That's what I want now too.

Workout totals: 6 miles

DAY 31

A Sad Day

The only easy day was yesterday.
—SEAL

New York City
31°
0800

I wake up on my own at 8:00 a.m. and the house feels different; the energy has changed.

I go to SEAL's room, but there's no SEAL. He's gone. The room is spotless, and the bed is perfectly made with military corners. You could bounce a quarter off it. Everything is *exactly* the way it was before he arrived. It's like he was never even here. Eerie.

When I walk into the kitchen, I see a note.

It's from SEAL.

No big sendoff. No big good-bye. No big anything. Just three words:

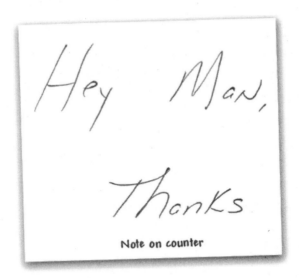

Note on counter

That's it. That's all he wrote. The guy woke me up at 5:00 a.m. for thirty days but didn't wake me up to say good-bye.

It starts to sink in that it's over. SEAL has returned to base.

Though SEAL left no trace in the bedroom, his fingerprints are all over the rest of the house. For example, every bedroom now has a fire extinguisher and a flashlight. Lazer, Sara, and I have full fire suits, in case we wake up one night and, God forbid, the place is an inferno. *And*, if the shit really hits the fan, behind our bar is an inflatable knapsack that turns into a life raft with oars and an attachable motor. It's there just in case some 9/11 shit happens. If anybody asks about it, I say what SEAL said to us: "It's our escape vehicle out of Manhattan, bitch." I also made a recent purchase at an outdoor furniture store in Atlanta, just in case I have to "camp out" on somebody.

SEAL also left an indelible mark on me. I've never been stronger, faster, or mentally tougher (take me to a frozen lake and I'll show you!). I can do a thousand push-ups in a day. I smoke the times I used to do around the Central Park Loop. I literally don't have an ounce of fat on me. But getting me in supreme shape was only a part of what SEAL did for me.

I have houses, a driver, fly privately. I have all of these things. SEAL has a military ID and cash. That's what he walks around with, just a backpack of belongings. He didn't want my life and I wanted his life. For starters, I'm going to simplify things. I'm going to try to get down to thirty items of clothing. I'm going through my closets and the extra shit in the garage and getting rid of stuff. I started deleting all of my emails, and it felt great. I started not answering people right away, and it felt fantastic.

SEAL clearly didn't want any part of our lives. I really admired how easy he lived his life. He didn't have to listen to others or have a team of people weigh in when making decisions. Part of that comes with the territory, and I get it. The simplicity that SEAL has is one of the most important things in life. He gets to do what he loves every day. He lives stress-free.

When SEAL broke both feet in the ultra-marathon with the twenty-thousand-foot climb, it wasn't the first time. He breaks his feet often when he runs grueling ultras. He has a hole in his aorta that surgeons can't seem to close. He's asthmatic.

And, he truly *hates to run.*

But he runs because he raises a lot of money for charity when he does to help the families of SEALs who died on the battlefield. One of the most emotional speeches I ever heard was Jimmy Valvano's at the ESPY Awards. Dying of cancer, with only months to live, he told the audience these important words. "Don't give up," he said. "Don't ever give up."

I hired SEAL because I wanted to get in the best shape of my life. I also hired him because I like the unexpected, and what better way to take a risk than having a Navy SEAL live with me for a month to train me? Finally, I hired him to get out of my routine, to shock the system, to mix things up so I could approach opportunities and challenges differently.

But I got much more than what I paid for.

"It's about protecting what you have," he said to me about being a SEAL. He might have been talking about defending democracy or freedom or saving us from terrorism. But I think he was talking about protecting something closer to home.

Now that SEAL is gone, I realize I don't need a lot of the crazy stuff in my life. These challenges I keep putting in front of myself to fulfill me. I'm not going to do any more of that. I'm staying put and focusing on the little things. I don't need manufactured adventures in my life to change me.

But maybe the most important thing I learned from SEAL was the level of appreciation he has for difficulty. The harder the training, the more courage it took to do and the more satisfaction was derived from it. SEAL taught me that you only get one shot at life and you should find out what's in your reserve tank. Coasting is for "pussies" as SEAL would say and it's when you dig deep that you feel the most alive. He lives his life that way. And some of that rubbed off on me.

EPILOGUE

A couple of months after SEAL moved out, Sara and I took a short vacation to the Bahamas. I invited SEAL to come down for a few days of R&R. It was going to be a quick trip, but I wanted to see if he was interested in joining us.

"Roger that," he said.

He brought *no luggage*, only his own bike and a stationary bike setup.

"I'm going to get a couple of hundred miles in," he said.

"On the island?"

"Nah, in my room."

We were there for three days, he put the PRIVACY sign on his doorknob, and he never left his room. The most beautiful setting in the world: girls, gambling, ocean the color of a Dodgers hat. He never went out. He just pushed his bed up against the wall so he could face the ocean and ride: Ocean Club, the Atlantis, twenty-seventh floor was SEAL's workout center. He said he was training for a bike ride across America.

One year later...

I'm in my office with Kish. The phone rings and she picks it up. She's smiling.

"It's for you," she says with her hand over the receiver.

"Who is it?" I whisper.

"SEAL," she whispers back.

"Hey, man. How are you?"

"Good," SEAL says.

"What's going on?"

"Just giving you a heads-up I'm in New York for some meetings today," he says.

"Cool," I say. "You wanna crash with us?"

"Nah, man, I don't want to impose on ya. Just wanted you to know I'm in town."

"Well, where are you going to stay?"

"I'm just going to sleep in Central Park," he says.

I look out the window of my office. It's snowing and my computer says fourteen degrees.

"Roger that," I say. "I'm thinking it's going to be seventy and sunny."

Day	Miles Run	Push-Ups	Pull-Ups	Sit-Ups	Burpees	Jumping Jacks	Box Jumps	Flutter Kicks	Fireman Carries
1	6	0	100	0	0	0	0	0	0
2	12	0	0	0	0	0	0	0	0
Totals (Days 1 - 2)	18	0	100	0	0	0	0	0	0
3	14.3	0	0	0	0	0	0	0	0
Totals (Days 1 - 3)	32.3	0	100	0	0	0	0	0	0
4	6	100	36	0	0	0	50	0	0
Totals (Days 1 - 4)	38.3	100	136	0	0	0	50	0	0
5	0	150	0	0	0	0	0	0	0
Totals (Days 1 - 5)	38.3	250	136	0	0	0	50	0	0
6	12	300	0	0	100	0	0	0	0
Totals (Days 1 - 6)	50.3	550	136	0	100	0	50	0	0
7	17	275	0	0	0	0	0	0	0
Totals (Days 1 - 7)	67.3	825	136	0	100	0	50	0	0
8	6	0	0	0	0	0	0	0	0
Totals (Days 1 - 8)	73.3	825	136	0	100	0	50	0	0
9	6	0	10	100	0	0	0	0	0
Totals (Days 1 - 9)	79.3	825	146	100	100	0	50	0	0
10	2	171	30	0	0	0	0	0	0
Totals (Days 1 - 10)	81.3	996	176	100	100	0	50	0	0
11 - 12	8	484	0	132	0	0	0	0	0
Totals (Days 1 - 12)	89.3	1480	176	232	100	0	50	0	0
13	8	200	0	0	0	800	0	0	0
Totals (Days 1 - 13)	97.3	1680	176	232	100	800	50	0	0
14	6	0	0	0	100	0	0	0	14
Totals (Days 1 - 14)	103.3	1680	176	232	200	800	50	0	14
15	8	350	0	0	0	0	0	0	0
Totals (Days 1 - 15)	111.3	2030	176	232	200	800	50	0	14

(continued)

Day	Miles Run	Push-Ups	Pull-Ups	Sit-Ups	Burpees	Jumping Jacks	Box Jumps	Flutter Kicks	Fireman Carries
16	17	0	0	0	0	0	0	0	0
Totals (Days 1 - 16)	128.3	2030	176	232	200	800	50	0	14
17	3	465	0	50	0	0	0	50	0
Totals (Days 1 - 17)	131.3	2495	176	282	200	800	50	50	14
18	0	364	30	0	0	0	0	100	0
Totals (Days 1 - 18)	131.3	2859	206	282	200	800	50	150	14
19	6	200	0	0	0	0	0	0	0
Totals (Days 1 - 19)	137.3	3059	206	282	200	800	50	150	14
20	8	400	0	550	0	0	0	0	0
Totals (Days 1 - 20)	145.3	3459	206	832	200	800	50	150	14
21	10	0	0	0	0	0	0	0	0
Totals (Days 1 - 21)	155.3	3459	206	832	200	800	50	150	14
22 - 23	16.1	700	0	0	0	0	0	0	0
Totals (Days 1 - 23)	171.4	4159	206	832	200	800	50	150	14
24	3.5	154	0	0	0	0	0	0	0
Totals (Days 1 - 24)	174.9	4313	206	832	200	800	50	150	14
25	9.5	775	0	125	0	0	0	0	0
Totals (Days 1 - 25)	184.4	5088	206	957	200	800	50	150	14
26	9.5	0	0	0	0	0	0	0	0
Totals (Days 1 - 26)	193.9	5088	206	957	200	800	50	150	14
27	3.5	1000	0	0	0	0	0	0	0
Totals (Days 1 - 27)	197.4	6088	206	957	200	800	50	150	14
28	8.5	300	0	0	0	0	0	0	0
Totals (Days 1 - 28)	205.9	6388	206	957	200	800	50	150	14
29	10.6	100	30	0	0	0	0	0	0
Totals (Days 1 - 29)	216.5	6488	236	957	200	800	50	150	14
30	6	0	0	0	0	0	0	0	0
Totals (Days 1 - 30)	222.5	6488	236	957	200	800	50	150	14

Acknowledgments

I have always been a team sports guy. All great teams have outstanding teammates that are good at their positions. This book would not have been possible without the hard work of my teammates: Jennifer Kish, Lisa Leshne, Turney Duff, Rick Flynn, Marc Adelman, Adam Padilla, Bryan Black, Erica Jaffe, Marq Brown, Johnny "Photo," Joe Holder, Deana Levine, Stella Brown, Page Luther, Chelsea Kardokus, Kate Hartson, and the entire Center Street staff. Without them there is NO WAY this book would have come to fruition.

This book would obviously not have been possible without the support of my amazing wife, who let this outrageous stuff go on under her very own roof. Honey, I will NOT jump in a frozen lake again (fingers crossed).

Last, I wanted to thank SEAL for investing thirty-one days of his life to live with our family. The lessons I learned extend far beyond fitness. Thank you.

Great teammates believe in each other.

Roger that!